CANADIAN MEDICAL LIVES

DAVID M. BALTZAN

Prairie Doctor

Verne Clemence

Series Editor: T.P. Morley, M.D.

Associated Medical Services, Inc.
&
Fitzhenry & Whiteside
1995

Fitzhenry & Whiteside
195 Allstate Parkway
Markham, ON L3R 4T8

Jacket design: Arne Roosman
Copy Editor: Nicholas Stephens
Typesetting: JayTee Graphics
Printing & binding: Best/Gagné Book Manufacturers Inc.

Fitzhenry & Whiteside wishes to acknowledge the generous assistance and ongoing support of **The Book Publishing Industry Development Programme** of the **Department of Communications, The Canada Council** and **The Ontario Arts Council.**

Care has been taken to trace the ownership of copyright material used in the text, including the illustrations. The author and publisher welcome any information enabling them to rectify any reference or credit in subsequent editions.

Canadian Cataloguing in Publication Data

Clemence, Verne, 1937–
David M. Baltzan, prairie doctor

(Canadian medical lives ; 19)
Includes bibliographical references and index.
ISBN 1-55041-177-2

1. Baltzan, David M. (David Mortimer), 1897-1983.
2. Internists – Canada – Biography. I. Hannah Institute for the History of Medicine. II. Series.

R464.B3C54 1995 610'.92 C95-931633-7

PRINTED IN CANADA

CANADIAN MEDICAL LIVES SERIES

The story of the Hannah Institute for the History of Medicine has been told by John B. Neilson and G.R. Paterson in *Associated Medical Services Incorporated: A History* (1987). Dr. Donald R. Wilson, President of AMS, and the Board of directors decided that the Institute should produce this series of biographies as one of its undertakings.

The first ten biographies can be obtained through the retail book trade, or from Dundurn Press Ltd., 2181 Queen Street East, Suite 301, Toronto, ON M4E 1E5, and Dundurn Distribution, 73 Lime Walk, Headington, Oxford, England OX3 7AD.

The second group of biographies, of which this is the eighth volume, can also be obtained through retail book stores, or from Fitzhenry & Whiteside, 195 Allstate Parkway, Markham, ON L3R 4T8.

Veteran prairie journalist and author, Verne Clemence's lifelong interest in medicine makes him well suited to write about David Baltzan, devoted medical practitioner and dyed-in-the-wool prairie man.

Clemence describes how intense intellectual curiosity led Baltzan to become one of the earliest internists in the region, and how an equally intense zeal led to the creation of a renowned medical clinic in Saskatoon.

Baltzan was also the confidant of Prime Minister Diefenbaker, and as a result served with distinction on the Hall Commission — the Royal Commission on Health Services — which led to the establishment of Canada's system of universal health care.

As Clemence reveals, his subject, both as a member of the Royal Commission and as a distinguished leader in his field, was no dissembler in either politics or medical practice, but a genuine straight shooter, Western style.

There is no shortage of meritorious subjects. Willing and capable authors are harder to acquire. The Institute is therefore deeply grateful to authors who have committed their time and skill to the series.

T.P. Morley
Series Editor
1995

CANADIAN MEDICAL LIVES SERIES

Dundurn Press:

Duncan Graham by Robert Kerr and Douglas Waugh

Bill Mustard by Marilyn Dunlop

Joe Doupe by Terence Moore

Clarence Hincks by Charles G. Roland

Francis Scrimger by Suzanne Kingsmill

Emily Stowe by Mary Beacock Fryer

R.G. Ferguson by C. Stuart Houston

Harold Griffith by Richard Bodman and Deirdre Gillies

Earle P. Scarlett by F.W. Musselwhite

Maude Abbott by Douglas Waugh

Fitzhenry & Whiteside:

William Boyd by Ian Carr

J.C. Boileau Grant by C.L.N. Robinson

R.M. Bucke by Peter A. Rechnitzer

William Henry Drummond by J.B. Lyons

Alan Brown by A.B. Kingsmill

Harold N. Segall by C.G. Roland

William R. Beaumont by Julian A. Smith

David M. Baltzan by Verne Clemence

CONTENTS

To Miriam

List of Illustrations

Acknowledgements

The greatest debt of gratitude for this book is, of course, owed to the subject himself, an individual of extraordinary accomplishments who left his world a great deal better than he found it. David's sons Marc and Richard took precious time from their busy medical practices to share information about their father, along with affectionate anecdotes of family life. Their respect for him and his legacy shines through in every word. One-time partner Harold Sugarman, former friends and associates Rose Rudd and Lorna Whelan and a few former patients kindly granted interviews. Invaluable assistance was also given by the library of the Canadian Medical Association Journal. The Saskatoon Jewish Community Centre, the Saskatchewan College of Physicians and Surgeons, the Royal College of Physicians and Surgeons, the Diefenbaker Centre and the Saskatoon Archives Board were all helpful. My daughter Crystal helped with interviewing and research and put in endless hours transcribing tapes. My wife Miriam is always my best editor, my son Greg an errand boy and computer assistant. My old journalist friend Pat O'Dwyer gave me good advice. I thank them all. Any inaccuracies left in this manuscript are, of course, my sole responsibility.

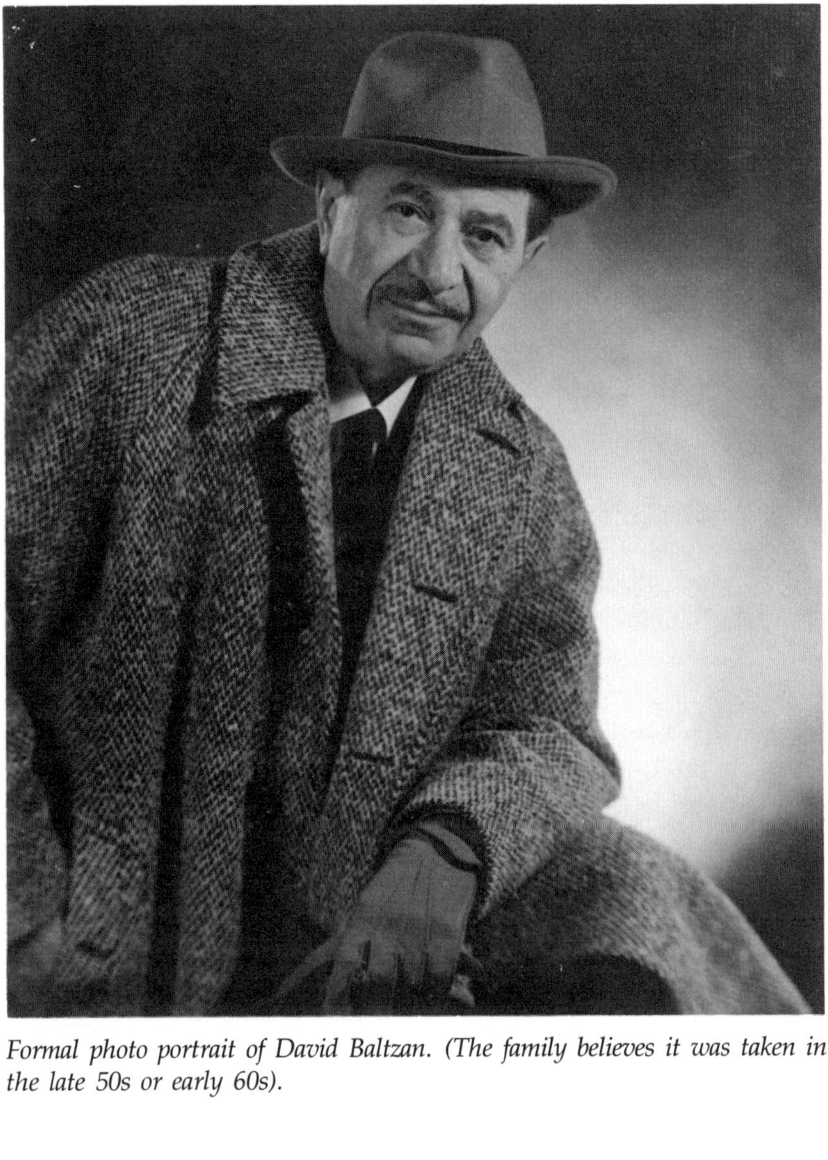

Formal photo portrait of David Baltzan. (The family believes it was taken in the late 50s or early 60s).

Introduction

When the distinguished internal medicine specialist David Baltzan retired from a 50-year career in Saskatoon in the mid-1970s, he was persuaded by family members and friends to give some thought to writing his memoirs. He got as far as preparing a skimpy outline before illness overtook his efforts. In consultation with a book editor friend, he had settled on a working title for his book: The Prairie Doctor. The words evoke images of dedicated family practitioners of the early years in isolated outbacks of the country, the doctors who went when and where they were called, winter and summer, and who thrived on self-reliance and an art founded as much on common sense as high science. While he was certainly the epitome of dedication, David Baltzan's practice was in an urban setting. What he did have in common with the family retainer physician of old was a vigorous skepticism that took nothing for granted, a capacity for improvisation when faced by uncertainty, and a life-long loyalty to the families he served.

In the title for his planned memoirs he left a clue about how he himself saw his career in medicine. To most who knew him and his work he seemed to stand for innovative diagnostic techniques and sophisticated medicine. But for much of his working life he must have felt that he was on the frontiers of the profession. It was David Baltzan who wondered out loud if there were links between smoking and heart disease long before others had raised the alarm; who stubbornly pursued the enigma of the cause of cyanosis in a case believed to be due to an anatomical abnormality of the heart until he found the true explanation was a genetic abnormality of blood chemistry; who looked for ways to make health care accessible to those unable to pay years before "medicare" had crept into the lexicon.

It was David Baltzan who placed the weight of his integrity behind early organ transplant programs while many others drew back from the ethical abyss they feared. The role of spiritual leader was one which eminently suited him and one he played in circles much wider than his own practice or family. A confidant, physician and friend to a prime minister; a scholar and teacher; a Jewish doctor who headed the most important committee in a Roman Catholic hospital for years and of whom it was said that the sisters "treated him like a bishop"; a doctor with roots in small town medicine who wrote off countless thousands in fees during the Depression; an academic with membership in scores of scientific societies, associations and groups — David Baltzan's honours, accomplishments and deeds are legendary. And yet, as his close friend Emmett Hall said in a terse eulogy, Baltzan "never looked for credit and did most of those things, and more, as a volunteer."

His is truly a life to celebrate. He was not able to write his own story. The Alzheimer's disease that took his life in 1983 prevented him from even starting to put it down in his own words. And because throughout his life he was a self-effacing individual whose copious energies were directed toward the needs of others, he was not given to recording his private thoughts as he went along; he left no diaries. What remains are some published professional papers, a few written archival records and the recollections of family members and others who knew the man and worked with him, or whose lives were touched by him in some way. All this is less than we want to know about the journey made by this quiet man, from a childhood on a southern Saskatchewan pioneer farm at the turn of the century, to the highest honours than can be accorded a medical practitioner. Lives such as his are reminders that the best in human achievement is never out of date.

— Chapter 1 —

The Hall Commission

DAVID BALTZAN turned down an assignment in June of 1965 to give a speech on the recently publicized report of the Royal Commission on Health Services, widely known as the Hall Report.[1]

"I declined the proposed topic because that report must stand or bend depending upon the forces which shape the future course of 'the best possible health services for all Canadians'," he told his audience, a national gathering of students in hospital administration attending a seminar at the University of Saskatchewan.[2]

Baltzan was 68 at the time and at the height of a prestigious career as a specialist in internal medicine, an educator and chief of the medical staff of a major hospital. His own Baltzan Clinic, an established referral centre in Saskatoon with an international reputation, was the realization of a life-long dream to have a family practice with his sons. He had just spent almost four gruelling years on the royal commission headed by his old friend Emmett Hall, former Chief Justice in Saskatchewan, and by then a judge of the Supreme Court of Canada.

Many months had been spent rushing from city to city in Canada for hearings, then hurrying home to take care of his responsibilities at the clinic. Commission members had also travelled extensively outside the country to assess health care systems worldwide. In subscribing to a consensus, Baltzan was often caught between the wishes of the majority on the commission and powerful forces from within the ranks of his own profession.

By mid-1965, no one would have blamed him if had he become fed up with the whole thing and abandoned it, especially since the question of implementation of the commission's findings was still up in the air.

Progressive Conservative Prime Minister John Diefenbaker had created the royal commission on health care in 1960, five years earlier. It would be early 1967 before legislation was passed in the House of Commons. By then the Diefenbaker Conservatives were in opposition, defeated by the Lester Pearson Liberals. The Liberals brought the bill into the House of Commons, but it was a further 18 months before it came into effect. It took almost a full decade for the initiative begun under Diefenbaker to reach fruition under Pearson.

Small wonder Baltzan steered away from the report in his talk to the students. Instead, he told them he would discuss the course of medicare programs "with the purpose of weaving the many loose threads into a tapestry depicting the panorama." As for the Hall Report, he said, the students would be better informed if they read the actual chapters of greatest interest to them in the book-length document.

Thus the students were treated to some of Baltzan's philosophical underpinnings, which in the end were in almost total accord with Emmett Hall's vision of a government-run health care service for Canada, affordable and universally accessible. That put Baltzan at odds with many in his profession and, reading between the lines of his 1965 speech, it almost seems as if he wanted someone to understand why he had reached certain conclusions.

He reminded the students that the commissioners had served as citizens-at-large and could not act in any way partial to "the many vested interests in any area." He admonished them as well to remember that "royal commissions recommend — governments amend!" He no doubt had a pretty good idea of the extent to which the recommendations were going to be altered as soon as the politicians got their hands on the report.

In his comments that day, Baltzan was pleading that political or bureaucratic manoeuvres not be allowed to go so far as to create an unworkable scheme. "Confidence in government could be greater if fear of vested political party interests was less," he observed.

His first point was that any system had to be guided by common sense, or "medisense," as he put it. "It means judging the subject as a whole, including its constituent parts, and not by any one constituent governing the whole. It means that which suits more people better, what greater good comes to all, how best to serve the sick and how more effectively preventive measures can be applied, and not what you or I alone favour."

Even the notion that everyone had a right to good health was fallacious, he pointed out, for the simple reason that such things as birth defects, hereditary afflictions, genetic flaws (he mentioned hemophilia, doubtless thinking back to his own haemoglobin discovery more than a decade earlier) and retardation are beyond human control. Rather, he said, everyone had a right to the *opportunities* for good health care.

As health care had grown more sophisticated in terms of knowledge and technology, it had also became more costly. The cost, said Baltzan, had reached such proportions as to cause "serious personal anxiety for the sick and their dependents." That led him neatly into the simple but very basic underlying issue of health care — the many models of voluntary systems attempted over the years had a fatal flaw: left to their own devices, too many citizens simply would not participate, leaving the financial burden primarily on those who needed to use the system. At the same time, the public, through newly compassionate governments, was paying for emergency treatment for those who had not subscribed to voluntary prepayment plans or private insurance and whose resources had been consequently wiped out by the expense of serious illness.

It was a point Baltzan returned to several times, but in different ways, during that speech. He warned that while government short-sightedness could be criticized for some inadequacies in health care, "the blame also rests with people at large, for lack of participation and inflictions upon governments to the point of surrender." More than most, he had closely observed various models of private health care over a lengthy period.

"As an eyewitness upon the scene from the beginning . . . I can safely put on record that the prepayment principle was the match that started the prairie fire which still rages," he said. He was referring, of course, to Saskatchewan's attempts to create a government-run medicare system, the event that had actually spurred the Canadian Medical Association to pressure the federal government to conduct a top-level investigation into health care country-wide.

"In the beginning, it was 'Money-care' not 'Medicare'. The unpaid accounts bothered the debtors as well as the creditors, including the neighbourhood druggist.''

There was little altruism at the outset, he said. Then new forces came into play, with ''instalment purchasing and pay-as-you-go'' health plans. ''In medical socio-economics, this trend took shape in the form of pay-before-you-get-sick.''

Baltzan harked back to 1936, when some members of the United Farmers Association in Saskatchewan and a few private citizens pooled their resources to pay when sickness struck. It was a system, in fact, which he had helped organize. He said only that the originators were encouraged and assisted ''gratuitously by a few doctors,'' adding that those pioneers had not yet come upon the word ''prepayment.'' The scheme functioned as a private, non-profit, ''friendly'' group and was officially incorporated in 1939 as the Saskatoon Medical Mutual and Hospital Association.

Thereafter, prepaid systems spread throughout the country, pushed by doctor-sponsored plans. Baltzan watched them all and participated in some. He concluded that they paved the way for a more comprehensive system; they proved there was a demand; they offered broad protection; they advanced the non-profit model. But in the end, the prepayment systems also proved that ''the healthy and the indifferent did not join and so the costs were too high for the sick alone to bear; they proved an arbitrary dividing line could not be established between low income and higher income groups.'' The solution implemented by operators of many of the successful prepayment schemes was to deny enrolment to individuals but accept only groups — usually large ones such as employees of a company — thus enforcing the insurance principle of spreading the load.

At the very end of his speech, in a short section headed ''Deduction,'' Baltzan did, finally, seem to discuss the Hall Report.

''Canadians want universal insurance coverage: no one left out; comprehensive health services; no half diagnosis and incomplete treatment offering more than 'minimal services' or only 'essential services'; freedom for self-governing professions and freedom for patients to recognize authorities where they may find the best results, including the right to collect the costs for sickness in the amount paid under *any* universal comprehensive insurance plan; none has to be Crown corporation in the operational sense; to endure, the plans must be secured by the maintenance of an elaborate supportive structure.''

* * *

Baltzan had revealed as much about himself as he had the history of prepaid medical schemes as he sketched the ''panorama'' of medical care programs that day.

No doubt John Diefenbaker himself had heard some of the same common sense argued by David Baltzan — his friend, and the doctor to whom he entrusted the welfare of his closest family members when they needed care. The Prime Minister insisted that, whoever else Emmett Hall wanted on the commission he was to head, it was mandatory that Baltzan be invited to serve.

More than 30 years later, Hall looked back on the creation of the commission and told one of his favourite stories:

> The Canadian Medical Association went to Diefenbaker in December of 1960 and urged him to appoint a commission to look into it (health care) because of all the hell that was going on here in Saskatchewan. I was chief justice of the trial division at that time and I was presiding over a trial (in Regina), and I got a message from Diefenbaker that he wanted to talk to me on the phone. After I adjourned the trial we talked and he told me about it, that the medical people were pressing him to do this. He wanted to know what I thought. I thought it was pretty good and I said, 'Well, it sounds like a good idea.'
>
> He says, 'Okay, I'll be in touch with you.'
>
> That was about 11 or 12 in the morning and I went over to the Assiniboia Club for lunch. The news was on, saying that I'd been appointed chairman of the commission.[3]

Hall recalls that he heard nothing more from Diefenbaker for several months. Then, after the CMA had held its annual meeting in late May or early June and ''pounded the hell out of the Old Man for this commission,'' he (Hall) was called to Ottawa. Diefenbaker gave him a long list of names from which to choose the members of his commission.

''Choose anybody, but choose one man, Dave Baltzan,'' Hall was told.

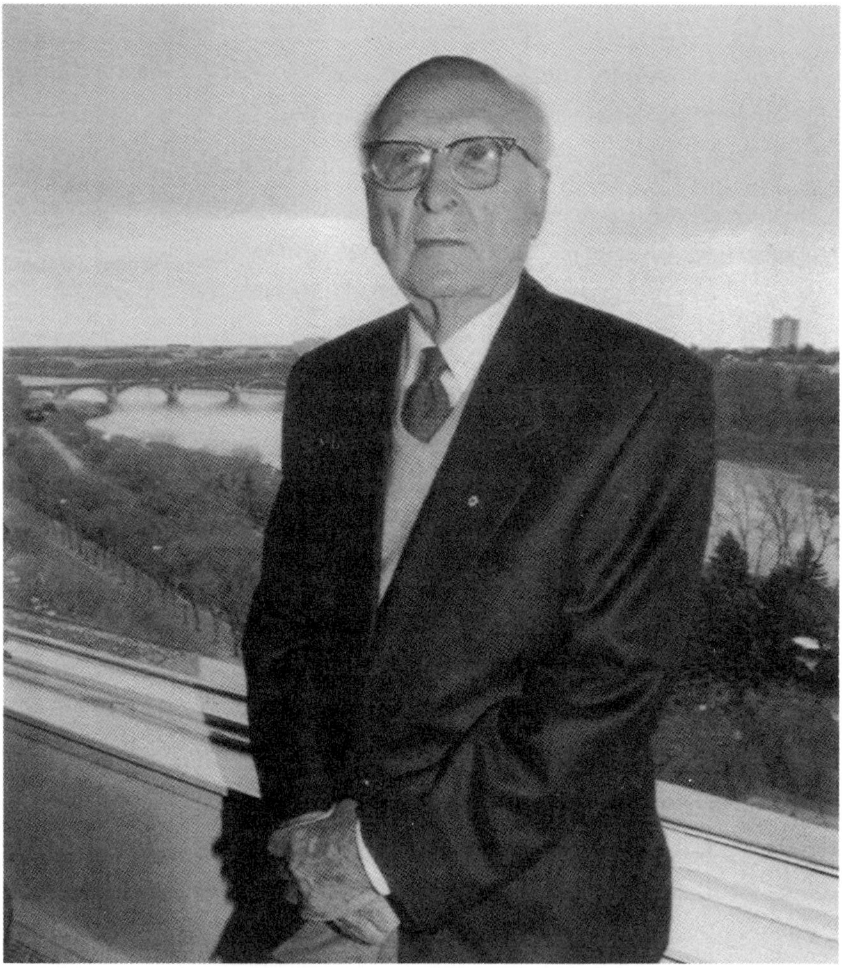

Emmett Hall, October 1993. Courtesy Saskatoon StarPhoenix

"I said, 'Oh, hell, that suits me perfectly'."

Hall spent the next few months in frantic activity. Along with the job of creating the commission, consulting with the members and setting an agenda for cross-country hearings, he accepted the appointment of Chief Justice of the Court of Appeal in Saskatchewan. He called it a "part-time job" years later, saying that was the only way he could handle the commission job at the same time. But he still maintained a hectic schedule during those years. And before his work with the health care commission was completed, he was elevated again, this time to Justice of the Supreme Court of Canada. Again, he cited a workload substantially less than the Supreme Court justices would face two decades later as the factor that made it possible for him to hold down two demanding positions at the same time.

Along with Baltzan who, among other attributes of value to the task at hand, was past president of the Saskatchewan Medical Association, Hall appointed Alice Girard, past president of the Canadian Nurses' Association; Arthur Van Wart, past president of the Canadian Medical Association; Cecil L. Strachan, a London, Ontario, dentist; O.J. Firestone, a wealthy Ottawa economist, and Wallace McCutcheon, a Toronto life insurance executive, founder of the Argus Corporation and a business partner of E.P. Taylor. McCutcheon resigned after attending hearings for less than a year, having been appointed to the Senate and the federal cabinet.

The commission began its hearings in September 1961. By the end of March 1963, the members had heard from individuals and special interests in St. John's, Halifax, Charlottetown, Fredericton, Quebec City, Montreal, Toronto, Ottawa, Winnipeg, Regina, Edmonton, Vancouver, Victoria and Whitehorse. In all, 406 submissions had been received. Representatives of the commission also visited the United Kingdom, France, Holland, Sweden, Switzerland, Austria, Italy, the United States, the Soviet Union, Australia and New Zealand.

The commission's mandate was exceedingly broad. The terms of reference instructed Hall to "inquire into and report upon the existing facilities and the future need for health services for the people of Canada and the resources to provide such services, and to recommend such measures, consistent with the constitutional division of legislative powers in Canada, as the Commissioners believe will insure that the best possible health care is available to all Canadians and, in particular, the Commissioners shall inquire into and report upon:

(a) the existing facilities and methods for providing personal health services including prevention, diagnosis, treatment and rehabilitation;
(b) methods of improving such existing health services;
(c) the correlation of any new or improved program with existing services;
(d) the present and future requirements of personnel to provide health services;
(e) methods of providing adequate personnel with the best possible training and qualifications for such services;
(f) the present physical facilities and the future requirements for the provision of adequate health services;
(g) the estimated cost of health services now being rendered to Canadians, with projected costs of any changes that may be recommended;
(h) the methods of financing health care services;
(i) the methods of financing any new or extended programs which may be recommended;
(j) the relationship of existing and any recommended health care programs with medical research and the means of encouraging a high rate of scientific development in the field of medicine in Canada;
(k) the feasibility and desirability of priorities in the development of health care services; and
(l) such other matters as the Commissioners deem appropriate for the improvement of health services.''

Hall recalls that David Baltzan attended every hearing the commission held in Canada. As well, he spent about two weeks looking at the system in the Soviet Union, studied the American system closely and, Hall believes, he also travelled to Sweden to acquaint himself with health care there. According to Hall, Baltzan reported to the commission that the Swedish system was the best he had seen.

Although the commission became a household word in later years, it did much of its work in the early 1960s in relative obscurity. Hall recalls the heavy schedule and the fact that the members received only $100 a day over and above their expenses. As a judge of the Supreme Court, Hall himself could take no stipend of any kind. He says they all had to reach into their own pockets, Baltzan in particular, since the expenses of his practice went on. Richard took a year off from his training to come home and help out.

David's son Marc had joined the practice by that time and he also recalls his father's busy schedule. He says David was "very interested" in the whole process, answering, as it did, so many of the concerns he had had over the years.

"He strongly believed that everyone in society should have access to care. When you go back and look at the meticulous report they put together, it can almost be seen as the founding of medical economics."

Both Marc Baltzan and Emmett Hall say the commission did its work over all those months virtually without conflicts among its members. For the most part, such official records as there are confirm the accuracy of such recollections, although there is at least one account which suggests a few tense moments towards the end of the process. In *Emmett Hall: Establishment Radical*, former Saskatchewan journalist Dennis Gruending wrote that in January 1965 it came time to put the finishing touches to the second volume of the commission's report.

Baltzan had deep misgivings. The medical profession had punished him and Van Wart after the first volume was viewed as a proposal on a national scale for a system very close to the one implemented in Saskatchewan. The insurance industry had also reacted with hostility. Doctors had vented their collective spleen on Baltzan and Van Wart in private at a CMA meeting in Vancouver, and Wallace McCutcheon, a former commission member, even gave the two a dressing down in public in the presence of peers.[4] Some members of the Conservative caucus were also critical, though Diefenbaker himself pronounced it to be a "great social document."[5]

Hall did a supreme job of selling the report, however, especially considering the fact that it was, in effect, the CMA's worst nightmare. It went far beyond expectations to recommend, essentially, Saskatchewan medicare writ large. Among other things, it called for a universal, compulsory, tax-financed program, as well as a program to pay for prescription drugs, free dental care for welfare recipients, pregnant women and children under 18, eye care, fluoridation of water, care for disabled and mentally retarded children, better air-ambulance service and six new medical schools in the country. The job of convincing doubters was made easier with McCutcheon no longer part of the commission.

Ironically, Baltzan ultimately was the only holdout. He made a last-minute request that doctors practising outside the plan be allowed to bill their patients, who could in turn collect from the provincial medical insurance commission — the same clause the doctors had won in the Saskatoon Agreement, which ended the Saskatchewan doctors' strike in 1962 (in which, it should be noted, the Baltzans did not withdraw their services).

The other commissioners refused to support Baltzan's plea, especially since he had previously indicated agreement with the consensus (albeit reluctantly and after lengthy discussions with Hall). Still, with the report already at the printers, he again raised the issue, saying if the rest of the commission would not go along with his wish, he wanted such a clause included in the report in his name alone. He reminded Hall and the others in a telegram that he had believed all along that the second volume of the report was to offer an opportunity to spell out details. In the end, the printers were called in on overtime and the second volume was amended to include Baltzan's clause under an asterisk.

The change was not at the front of the report, as Baltzan had asked, but rather was on the last page of text. Its location was not the issue to David Baltzan, however. His son Richard remembers the ''asterisk'' skirmish as one of great importance to his father.

The disagreement was minuscule in comparison to the overall importance to the country of the Hall Commission report. As its architects, Baltzan, Hall and the other commissioners redrew Canadian society and created for the country a progressive, compassionate image, the shape of which, though frequently attacked, is bold enough to have survived the worst of times.

Chapter 2

Coming to Canada

DAVID MORTIMER Baltzan was born in 1897 in what was then Bessarabia, a province of Tsarist Russia. Bessarabia, acquired by Russia from Turkey in 1812, was annexed by Romania in 1918.

In 1924, the Soviet Union took part of the country when it established the Moldavian Autonomous Soviet Socialist Republic on the eastern bank of the Driester River. In 1940, that territory was merged with Romanian-speaking districts of Bessarabia, forming the Moldavian S.S.R. Now Moldova, the country declared independence in 1991.

Some family members believe David Baltzan's place of birth was a small town named Baltz, near Kishinev, the capital city of modern day Moldova. However, David's uncle, Jacob Baltzan, in a memoir about early life in Canada[1], refers to Leova as the Baltzan home town. Either way, Kishinev was the principal urban centre, and a cousin of the Saskatoon Baltzans, Leonid Baltzan, is today editor of the Jewish newspaper there.

Both Jacob Baltzan's memoirs and family history known to Baltzan family members establish that the pre-1900 family in Bessarabia was part of the wealthy landowning class. Jacob refers to his brother Moishe (David's father) as "a friendly, practical, successful salesman who had dealt in grain, wood, wool, sheep and other chattels" in the old country. The family home was a walled estate. The Baltzans had their own rabbi and were careful followers of Jewish practices and traditional ways.

In his writings, Jacob compared his homeland — "the beautiful, warm Bessarabia district . . . where peasants make wine and pick fruits and harvest corn 'til very late in the year" — to the cold, inhospitable Canada he first saw on his autumn journey from New York to Qu'Appelle.

* * *

Bessarabia, having been fought over for generations and having had a variety of different political masters, was a cultural crossroads of sorts. Russian, Romanian and Ukrainian influences were all strong. There was also an Asian presence. Permeating all was the anti-Semitism that swept eastern Europe in the late 19th century. It was becoming an inescapable factor for the Baltzans, as it was for Jews of all classes, Romanian, Ukrainian and Russian alike.

With Russia expanding eastward, war with Japan eventually broke out and the Tsar began to conscript Jewish farmers and merchants. It was during this time that many residents of the area began to look abroad for new opportunities and new homes.

One such was Moishe Baltzan. It is believed he left his family in Bessarabia and joined others in a sea voyage to North America. He and his companions went first to North Dakota in the northern United States, where they heard of a Jewish colony being established in the Qu'Appelle Valley in Canada. Free land was being offered to Russian Jews under the auspices of Sir Thomas Lipton, of Lipton Tea fame. Moishe headed north and, early in 1903, obtained a quarter section near what later became the town of Lipton, about 60 kilometres northeast of Regina. Though his own tenure was relatively brief, that same piece of land is still owned by Baltzan descendants.

Moishe's brother Jacob arrived in New York in 1904 and embarked on a journey of several days by train and horse-drawn wagon to join Moishe at the Qu'Appelle colony. He found a dispirited group of settlers, a mixture of Romanians and Russians, peasants and aristocrats, who didn't get on and who had made little progress in almost a year of trying to farm. Some lived in dugouts, others were using sod for temporary shelters. Jacob was not impressed and chided his brother and others for what seemed to be a lacklustre start. He looked in vain for signs of a Jewish school, or any central gathering place. Little or no land had been broken. Some of the original settlers had already lost heart and had gone elsewhere in search of better lives.

Jacob concluded that Moishe, who was in partnership with a brother-in-law, was enthusiastic about the new land, but out of his element. Neither Moishe nor Jacob had ever actually laboured on the land before. They had much to learn and would make many mistakes before they would be able to bring their families to Canada to live in respectable houses. And no matter how comfortable their new homes would become, they would never again enjoy the opulence they had known in Bessarabia.

Nevertheless, learn they did, and in February 1905, Moishe travelled to Winnipeg to greet his newly arrived wife Yetta and sons David and Harry.

Jacob had intended to stay in Canada only for the winter of 1904-05. After helping to construct a substantial new house on Moishe's land, however, and after gardens had been planted and crops sown, he, like Moishe, had acquired a deeper appreciation and understanding of the new world. Where before he was moved to expressions of dismay at the sight of vegetables left to rot, now he realized that there were not yet the same ready markets in this vast young land as there were in the more densely populated area of Bessarabia where he had lived before. He decided to put his Bessarabian holdings up for sale and bring his own family over.

In the months ahead, the brothers' newfound enthusiasm and determination were tested to the limit. The Baltzans endured the horrors of a raging prairie fire, the heavy slog of wet prairie clay, the sudden destructive power of a hailstorm and the piercing cold and deep snow of a western Canadian winter.

Not only did they have to learn how to make tools and build everything by hand, but they also had to come to grips with the questionable economics of homestead farming. They wisely came to the conclusion that their best chance at success lay in mixed farming. Tenuous markets and the vagaries of weather made an all-wheat operation too risky for their liking. Similarly, reliance on cattle alone would have exposed them not only to the ravages of the weather, but also to the risk of disease and injury to their herds. They bought cattle in small numbers and got full value in dairy products and meat for their own use and sold the excess when they could.

Even with astute management, however, Jacob writes in one passage of the despair he felt after drought took his crops and he had no money. He actually talked to his wife about leaving the farm. Finally, without telling her, he took a piece of silverware to town to sell for a little cash. When he picked up his mail in town, he was amazed to find that his family back in Bessarabia had sent him a substantial sum of money just in time. Little could he know that almost a century later, prairie farmers would still be looking for off-farm windfalls in order to be able to stay farming for another few years.

Jacob didn't write much about what farm life was like for his nephews David and Harry. In one passage, subtitled 'The Daily Routine,' he describes a typical day:

> Early in the morning Abie, Sam and I milked the cows. The milk was taken from us and delivered in pails to the milkhouse where my brother [Moishe] did the separating while reading the *Tangenblatt* or the *Americaner* [Jewish newspapers of that time]. Emptying the pails were my nephews, David [now D.M. Baltzan of Saskatoon], and Harry [owner of Crescent furniture in Edmonton] . . .

The reference to the milkhouse is especially interesting, since the structure served also as a library and study centre. Both brothers, Moishe in particular, were scholarly. As noted earlier, when Jacob arrived at the Qu'Appelle colony, he lamented that there were no facilities for study or discussion groups. Clearly the intellectual side of their lives was accorded a high priority, so they took the unusual step of creating a resource centre for reading and study in the midst of their farm work, where, as Moishe was portrayed above, they let no opportunity go to waste. Moishe, in fact, was a linguist, possibly speaking as many as seven languages. He was also a Hebrew scholar of note and a skilled writer, as was Jacob, who mentions at one point that he submitted regular articles to a periodical of the time.

Jacob's memoir is not dated. It seems obvious, however, that it was written some years after he had left the farm, possibly when he was living in Edmonton, where he moved after operating a store for some years at Govan, Saskatchewan. He explained at the outset that he was writing about those early years because the Jewish Press had not done justice to the many Jewish families who had not stuck with their farms in the original colony.

Presumably, in Jacob's view the true nature of the hardships experienced by many, particularly individuals such as he and Moishe, who had no previous experience, were not being adequately explained. If that was his purpose he served it well, though his paper ends rather abruptly with the thought that there is much more to come, and that he plans to get back to writing more at some future date. If he did, the material is nowhere to be found.

Reading between the lines, and hearing family lore from Moishe's grandsons, it is safe to conclude that neither of the Baltzan brothers was well suited to farming, even though Jacob's memoir suggests they did achieve a good deal by teaching themselves as they went along.

Either way, by about 1908 both had moved on.

Moishe took his family to Saskatoon, in part at least out of concern for his sons' education. Beyond that, his natural skills appeared to be in business, and he prospered in the city after starting up the Saskatchewan Hide and Fur Company.

Young David was dispatched to Princess Alexandria school, then to the Saskatoon Collegiate Institute, where he graduated. Family lore has it that among other exploits at that school, he won an oratory contest against classmate John George Diefenbaker, a man who in later life became as well known for his oratory as Baltzan was for his medical expertise.

David went into the hide and fur business with his father for a time, but eventually decided to study medicine. He started by attending medical school in Alberta. Apart from a recollection by a long-time office clerk[2] that she once heard him say that the things he most cared about were the practice of medicine and his family, there is no precise record of why he chose the medical path. As far as is known now, he was the first in his family to become a doctor.

World War I interrupted his plans. He did not see service overseas, but spent his time in the medical corps in Calgary. With the war over, David decided to go to McGill University in Montreal to complete his medical training; he graduated in 1920. The David Baltzan of the McGill class of that year was a somewhat more worldly specimen than the strictly raised Jewish youth of the old Lipton farm days. Classmate Harold Segall, in a eulogy to his great friend published in 1983,[3] recalled some high jinks from student days.

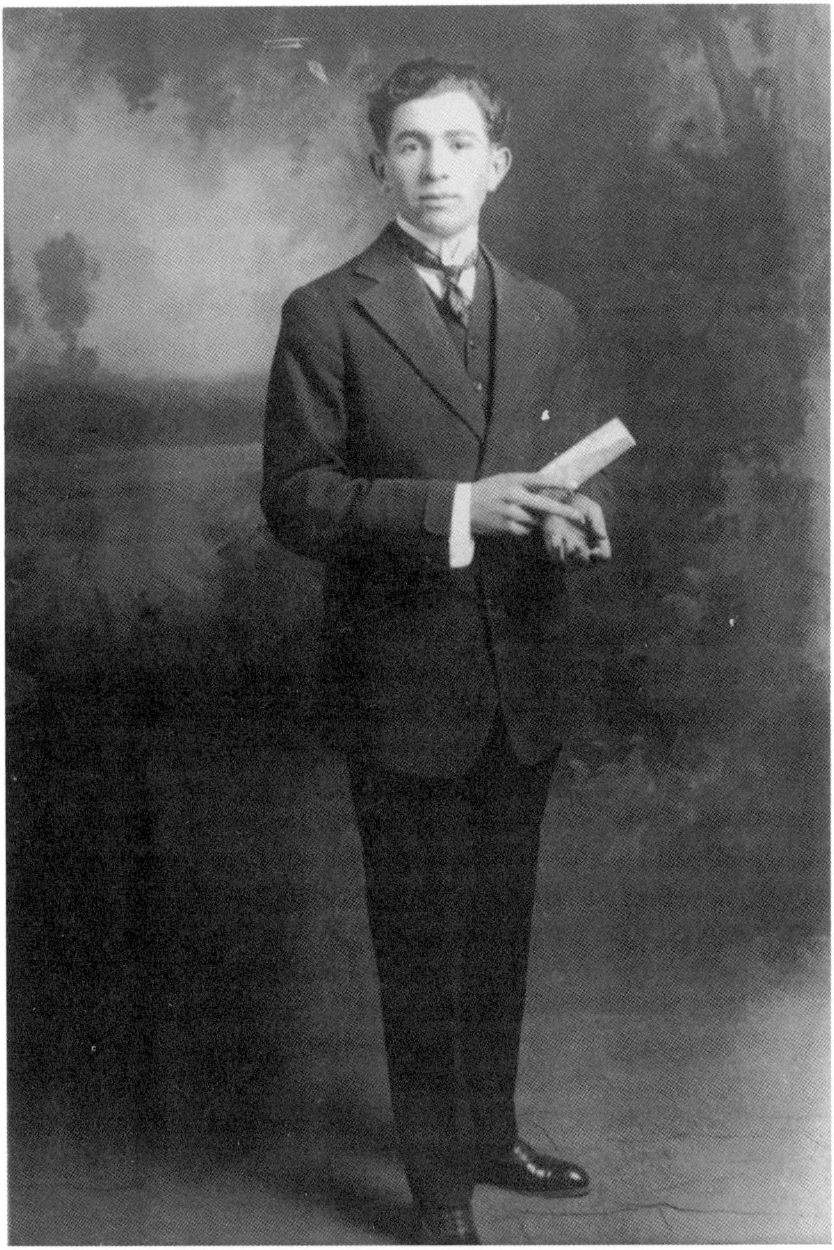

A young David Baltzan holding oratory prize. (This was the competition in which David reportedly defeated schoolmate John Diefenbaker).

After the final exam, Baltzan and Segall planned to celebrate the big day with a few other students. Segall was late arriving. When he finally showed up, David told him how he had bet another friend that he could outdrink him. "Dave told me about the bet and bid me to look at the challenger, who was sound asleep upstairs in his bedroom."

Things were not at all funny after graduation, however. Baltzan found, as did others in that anti-Semitic time, that it was difficult for a Jewish doctor to get an internship in Montreal. Nevertheless, he did manage to intern for a time at Montreal General, then went on to complete his practical experience at New York Lying-In Hospitals. He returned to Canada for a short period in 1921-22 as a junior associate in a general practice.

Baltzan decided in the mid-1920s to specialize in internal medicine. A recollection by another former office staffer may offer a clue as to why David made this choice. She says he once told her[4] that he had planned on a career in obstetrics, but when he lost a baby the experience so traumatized him that he vowed never to perform another delivery. The decision meant several years of postgraduate study in Edinburgh, London, England, Vienna and, finally, at Johns Hopkins in Baltimore.

He returned to Canada upon completion of his studies and in 1928 was offered a teaching post at the University of Alberta in Edmonton. He opted instead to come back to Saskatoon. He was married by then to Rose Cristall, the daughter of a wealthy Edmonton real estate family with its roots in Oxbow, Saskatchewan. There is some speculation[5] that David returned to Saskatoon because he wanted to be independent and freed from the influence of his in-laws. However, he explained to a newspaper reporter[6] years later that he chose Saskatoon because he was offered a clinic of his own by a medical group then in business in the city. The clinic failed to materialize, but David set up his own practice, fired by the need he saw at the time for modern innovations in internal medicine.

He was joined in the practice by an American laboratory technician he had met at Johns Hopkins, Wally Coleman. Eyebrows were raised when the two set up shop. Not only was Baltzan the first internist in the province, but the lab they set up was also a first. In a memo he wrote in 1965,[7] Baltzan recalled the reception he got from the medical establishment at the time:

> The status of what was to be known as Internal Medicine is illustrated by the greeting I received from our General Practitioner

> when I returned from Europe. 'What is this nonsense I hear about your plan not to do any surgery, and how can you expect a livelihood without an occasional appendectomy, haemorrhoidectomy . . .?'

Baltzan didn't waver. The upstart left surgery to others — and instead advanced medical practice in Saskatchewan by buying a portable electrocardiograph (ECG), using it in his office and taking it to hospitals until they acquired their own machines several years later. He and Coleman bought an X-ray machine as well. It was among the earliest — and possibly even the first — X-ray machine to be used in the province.

The response from medical colleagues continued to be one of perplexity. Surgery was king. Cutting was curing. Surgeons made the big incomes and had the prestige. Why would anyone do all that postgraduate work abroad and then come home and not operate? Even if he would not operate, would he not at least administer anaesthetics?

Baltzan's reply was that he had no intention of doing either; he intended to build a practice by concentrating on diagnostic internal medicine.

In spite of predictions that he couldn't possibly make a go of such a practice, he created the Baltzan clinic, persuaded his three sons to join him in it, and stayed actively involved himself for an incredible 50 years.

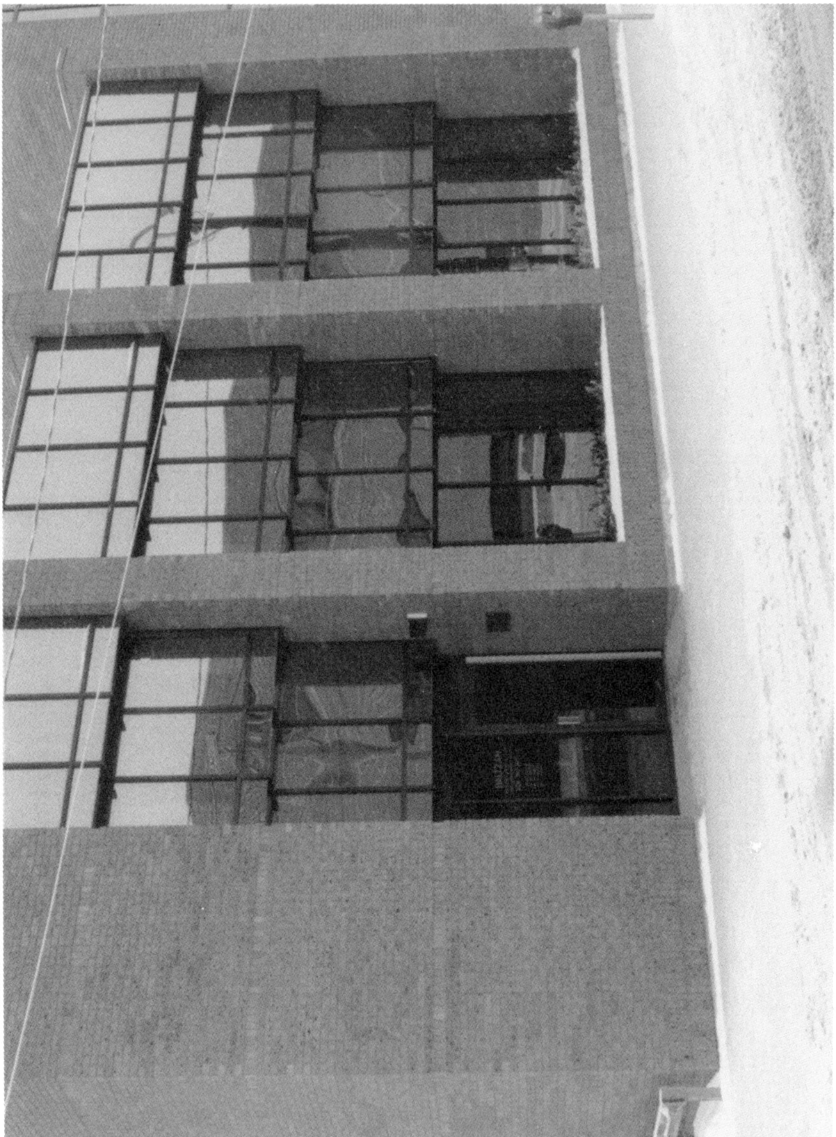

Baltzan Associate Medical Clinic. Photo courtesy Miriam Clemence

Chapter 3
Starting a Practice

TO START a new medical practice requires a certain amount of sacrifice, even under modern conditions. It took a good deal more back in pre-Depression Saskatoon, especially if the practice was to be limited to the new specialty of internal medicine, as was the case with David Baltzan's venture.

Internists were virtually unknown in western Canada in those days. Indeed, in the minds of many lay persons the word itself suggested "intern," which was thought by most to mean a doctor who was still learning the trade by working in a hospital. In fact, the opposite was true. The medical sleuths who could hang out their shingles as bona fide internists were doctors who had studied anatomy and diseases to a much greater extent than the general practitioners in whom most people had such unlimited faith. But internists were a misunderstood lot, and still are, judging by what many still apparently believe. Lewis Thomas, for example, president of the Memorial Sloan-Kettering Cancer Institute, in an essay in the *New Yorker* magazine in 1974, wrote:[1]

> The great secret, known to internists and learned early in marriage by internists' wives, but still hidden from the general public, is that most things get better by themselves.

If only that were true!

For the struggling new Baltzan medical practice, it was a matter of convincing other doctors to refer cases to him, and of appealing to the general public to use his services. And despite the prejudices, success was not long in coming — though by the nature of the specialty, Baltzan inevitably found himself burdened with the most difficult problems of the day.

All too often it was not possible to follow a correct diagnosis with effective treatment.

Before the days of open chest surgery, most heart and lung diseases were beyond help. Acute kidney failure was fatal. No treatment was available for cancer, other than radical (and often mutilating) surgery.

In daily contact with such life-threatening ailments, it is small wonder David Baltzan's talent for study and research came to the fore. He began to compile statistics from his practice and to publish his conclusions. The result made for an impressive body of work in the Journal of the Canadian Medical Association alone, where over 20 of his articles were published during his years of practice.

Building a practice from scratch meant long, arduous hours, at times with minimal reward and a discouragingly high rate of loss among patients. Medical practices were affected by the distances many country patients had to travel for treatment. The difficulties of getting to Saskatoon from outlying areas often meant health problems went unattended until they were beyond medical help.

In those early days, too, the area Baltzan served was only partly modernized. Most people lived without such amenities as indoor plumbing and sanitary sewage disposal. By modern standards, the general population lacked nutritional knowledge and was ignorant of the basics of personal and public health.

Nevertheless, there was an aura of adventure and hope in the undertaking.

The late Rose Rudd — she was Rose Collins then — worked for David Baltzan when he first practised after completing his studies at McGill. She was among the first office assistants the young doctor ever hired, working in the office with Baltzan and one other doctor in the 1920s. At age 90, looking back to those days, she remembered that office as something of a multi-cultural miracle.[2] There was Baltzan, the Romanian

Jew, herself, of Irish catholic stock, and a French doctor whose name she could not recall, "... and we all got along extremely well."

In the two years or so Rose worked in the Baltzan office, she came to admire the young doctor, and hinted that a romance might have bloomed under different circumstances. She recalled[3] with a chuckle that in the end David married a woman whose first name was also Rose, but the differences in religious backgrounds had ruled out anything other than friendship between doctor and clerk. They all "laughed and joked a lot," she said.

It was Rose who recalled Baltzan's story about his losing the baby and deciding against obstetrics — all part of his decision to study further and to specialize.[4] In any case, what she saw of David Baltzan at work convinced her of his talent. As long as he practised, he was her doctor; after he left active practice, she consulted his sons. Donald, the surgeon of the Baltzan group, performed life saving surgery on her in 1986, only two years before his own untimely death at 56 from cancer. And whenever she needed a referral to a specialist, she made sure it was to another Baltzan doctor, internist Richard.

* * *

Business picked up as Baltzan's reputation spread. Among other things, he accepted the job of first medical director at the Saskatoon Cancer Clinic, his main responsibility there being to examine the patients. Since cancer was still to all intents and purposes untreatable unless there was an operable tumour, one of his sad tasks was to try and predict for families how much time was left to terminal patients.

But there were also triumphs. A pre-school age child by name of John Chrones, for example, who would later become a successful Saskatoon restaurateur, was a beneficiary of David Baltzan's early treatment methods. Chrones was badly burned when hot wax spilled on one leg below the knee during play with a group of other children.[5] The Chrones's family doctor said amputation was the only answer, that the burn was too severe to heal and gangrene would set in. His parents, reluctant to give permission for the operation, heard of "this up-and-coming young doctor," Chrones recalls, and Baltzan was called in.

Understanding how tragic it would have been for the child and the family if the limb were lost, the young doctor tried what was then an unconventional treatment. After lengthy therapy, the burn healed and the leg was spared. Chrones still bears the livid scar and still recalls the painful time. Not surprisingly, when he needed bypass surgery some 60 years later, he turned again to the Baltzans.

The 1930s, of course, brought the years of the Great Depression. In that era of fee-for-service private practice, the tougher the times, the tougher the job of collecting. It was a problem that would stay with medical practitioners for many years, but the most severe time was in the last half of the 1930s.

Baltzan took on a partner in 1934. Harold Sugarman stayed with the practice for about 40 years. Many of his recollections are dimmed by the passage of time, but even the passing of so many years couldn't take away the vivid memories of patients with serious health problems and little or no money. The practice did not have enough funds to pay its staff on time, but Baltzan would not turn away patients, regardless of their ability to pay.[6]

Sugarman was just out of medical school when he joined the Baltzan Clinic as an employee.

"He (David) was very good to me. He gave me a real lift. I had no money. He helped me in every way possible and then we became partners in about a year's time."

The partnership, Sugarman recalls, was sealed with a handshake. There was never anything in writing until a few years before Sugarman retired, when younger partners came in who wanted written contracts.

The Dirty Thirties were hard for everyone. Sugarman remembers[7] a system that the rural municipalities of the day set up whereby municipal councils paid 25 percent of the fees for patients who came to the clinic but couldn't afford the full amount. Often the 25 percent was all the doctors received, since most people on farms in those days were without cash.

By his reaction to the hard times, Baltzan was instrumental in setting up the first medical care co-op. It was a system wherein participants pooled their premium money so that there would be something available for them if a medical emergency arose. The program was a forerunner to the larger Blue Cross MSI private insurance system, which Baltzan was also instrumental in getting started, along with Harold Sugarman who did much of the detail work. It was an entrepreneurial answer to the long-standing problem of physicians not being paid for their services.

The plan was widely subscribed until Saskatchewan implemented a government health care system in 1964. It remained popular in several other provinces for many years after that.

Sugarman's strongest recollection of his career with Baltzan is the ethical standards his partner upheld. As a practitioner, he recalls, Baltzan was more thorough than anyone he had ever worked with. In his retirement years, he often looks back with great fondness to his association with the entire Baltzan family.

Another friend from that era was Emmett Hall. Long before he was appointed justice to the Supreme Court of Canada and commissioner on many federal and provincial inquiries, Hall was a struggling lawyer. Like his medical counterparts, he worked hard to keep his practice afloat. He had graduated from the University of Saskatchewan law college in 1919, and after practising in Humboldt, Wadena and Prince Albert, he accepted in 1927 an invitation to join a firm in Saskatoon. He became friends with Baltzan in 1930 when the two occupied offices on the fourth floor of what was then the Provincial Building, later the MacMillan Building.

In his 90s at the time of writing, Hall is a tall, imposing figure. A widower for many years, he lives alone in downtown Saskatoon less than a block from the Saskatoon Club. He is a gracious host, explaining that the spacious, well-appointed apartment that has been his home for many years was the choice of his late wife Isabel (Belle). She was captivated by the view from a large east-facing living room window that looks out over the South Saskatchewan river and a stretch of manicured grass that runs down to the water's edge. The Halls sold the house they originally owned in Saskatoon when Emmett was appointed to the Supreme Court and they moved to Ottawa.

The former high court justice is not given to small talk. His austere manner quickly disappears, however, when conversation turns to any current issue. He is well-informed and becomes particularly animated when talking about the latest controversy swirling around the country's system of health care delivery. It is a short step from there to the royal commission he headed — and thence to the topic of the interview, his relationship with his long-time friend David Baltzan.[8]

"We had virtually the whole fourth floor of the Provincial Building between us," Hall remembers.

The two saw each other daily. They discussed local and national issues and came to hold great respect for each other's views. When Hall, who was a mover and shaker in Roman Catholic circles, became chairman of the board of St. Paul's hospital (operated by the Grey Nuns), their relationship grew even closer. Baltzan, active in Saskatoon's Jewish community in those days, was medical director at the hospital.

''We had no problems of any kind,'' Hall says, looking back. ''In fact,'' he observes wryly, ''we could often accomplish things in a phone call that it takes the bureaucracy of the hospitals of today weeks to settle.''

Hall says the whole hospital, including the sisters themselves, depended on Baltzan a great deal for many years. As to the religious issue, Hall says it ''just never came up. If Baltzan said it, it was true. He had the full respect of the sisters, who treated him like a bishop.''

Hall also recalls that Baltzan managed to get along quite well with the business establishment in the city, something that was crucial at that time when private fund-raising was so important. Hall, of course, was frequently arguing cases in court. Whenever he could, he would have Baltzan give evidence about medical matters.

''He was highly regarded. What he said was gospel.''

Hall was impressed by something else about David Baltzan at that time.

''I don't know how he did it, but it was quite an accomplishment for a Jewish boy from rural Saskatchewan to turn up in McGill University Medical School.''

Hall's regard for and friendship with David Baltzan would come into play some years later when they both served on the Royal Commission on Health Services. Indeed, the experience probably was a true test of their camaraderie , since it brought them as close as they would come to real conflict. But that was still 20 years or so in the future.

* * *

As the 1930s gave way to World War II, the Baltzan medical practice grew steadily, with its founder ever more in demand in medical and non-medical circles alike.

During the war years, ''we worked like dogs,'' explained Lorna Whelan, office manager at the clinic for some ten years. The clinic had developed a tremendous referral business by that time and it was almost routine for the staff to work until the last patient had been seen, at seven or seven-thirty in the evening. The bad debt problem continued in those years too, with thousands of dollars being written off.

Lorna Whelan started work at the clinic early in the 1940s. She had been a patient for some years, had had surgery and had made frequent visits for post-operative tests.

''Finally,'' she recalls,[9] ''somebody said, 'Why don't you get a job there? It would be easier.' ''

So she did, and the relationship lasted for many years.

In the absence of other training facilities, Baltzan and his American lab partner Wally Coleman taught Whelan to be their lab technician, taking over as manager of the office when Coleman later returned to the States.

As with others who look back on Baltzan's practice, she recalls his compassion. There was the sad case of a woman from a farm near Saskatoon who was referred to the clinic. The woman was 32, with two young children. After her second pregnancy she had developed problems with varicose veins. A country doctor had performed a vein ligation in his office. The woman ended up with gangrene and the only way to save her life was to amputate both legs.

''So she went back to the farm in a wheelchair after three months, and when the file came out to me, there was a big goose egg where the charge was supposed to be.''

But Whelan also recalls how Baltzan could also be somewhat taciturn with patients.[10] He was not a man to make small talk, with the result that some elderly patients, especially, found him difficult to talk to. She remembers one woman standing at the counter outside Baltzan's private office, fuming.

Wanting to ask a series of questions, but intimidated by the doctor, she had written them all down, covering two sides of a small card. She was fuming because she realized when she came to the counter to pay her bill that she had forgotten to turn the card over and had asked only half the questions.

Whelan remembers Baltzan's high standards as well, and his preoccupation with staying abreast of medical developments. He subscribed to all the medical journals and read them thoroughly. She recalls, too, the hundreds of medical books Baltzan collected at his home, and how in his wife's absence he had the kitchen remodelled, taking half of it in the process to make a library for himself. Rose, apparently, was amazed — and not at all pleased.

Whelan also remembers a routine Baltzan followed every week. The office was open Saturdays, but he would leave to attend a noon discussion group at the Bessborough Hotel with several others, among them the president of the university and others from the intellectual establishment in the city.

"We never knew what time he would be coming to see his patients. Eventually he would stagger in, and I'd have all these people laid out on those hard examining tables . . ."

But she knew the stimulation of the group discussions was important to Baltzan and she cannot recall his involvement in much else of a recreational nature. Mostly, whatever he did was connected to work.

What now impresses Whelan about her former employer is the extraordinary amount of time and work he put in as a member of the Royal Commission on Health Services, for which, in her view, he has been given scant credit over the years.

"He did so much, and he believed in it so much."

She recalls some lighter moments, like the chat she had one day with a long-time patient. The woman mentioned that she had seen Whelan's boss at the summer resort at Waskesui a few weeks earlier, dressed in swimming trunks.

"Have you ever seen his legs? Forget it," the woman laughed.

Small in stature, David Baltzan did not possess an athletic physique. He enjoyed robust good health, however, and had an exceptional capacity for hard work.[11] For the most part, he was experienced as an intensely serious fellow, reading glasses perched on the end of his nose, head thrust forward, looking directly at whomever he was talking or listening to.

That is not to say that he was incapable of lighter moments. Whelan also recalls him as being fun at a party, where, Scotch and ginger ale in hand, he could be highly entertaining when he felt like it.

He could also be arrogant, she says, though she has nothing but fond memories of the years of hard work she put in at the clinic.

* * *

Like most men of his age David Baltzan smoked cigarettes until about 1940, when he switched to cigars or a pipe. Whelan remembers his pipe because she once gave it a thorough cleaning in the office sterilizer, hoping to remove its pungent odour.

Baltzan, of course, was not pleased and took pains to explain how he had spent years seasoning the pipe until it was just right.

He gave up all forms of tobacco some time later, perhaps mindful of the growing weight of evidence from his own clinical research about the harmful effects of smoking. Elsewhere, more formal research in the ensuing years confirmed the suspicions Baltzan had written about as early as 1933 concerning the possible link between smoking and heart disease.

That was among the earliest of many health issues he brought to the attention of the medical community as a result of his lifelong habit of careful observation and record keeping.

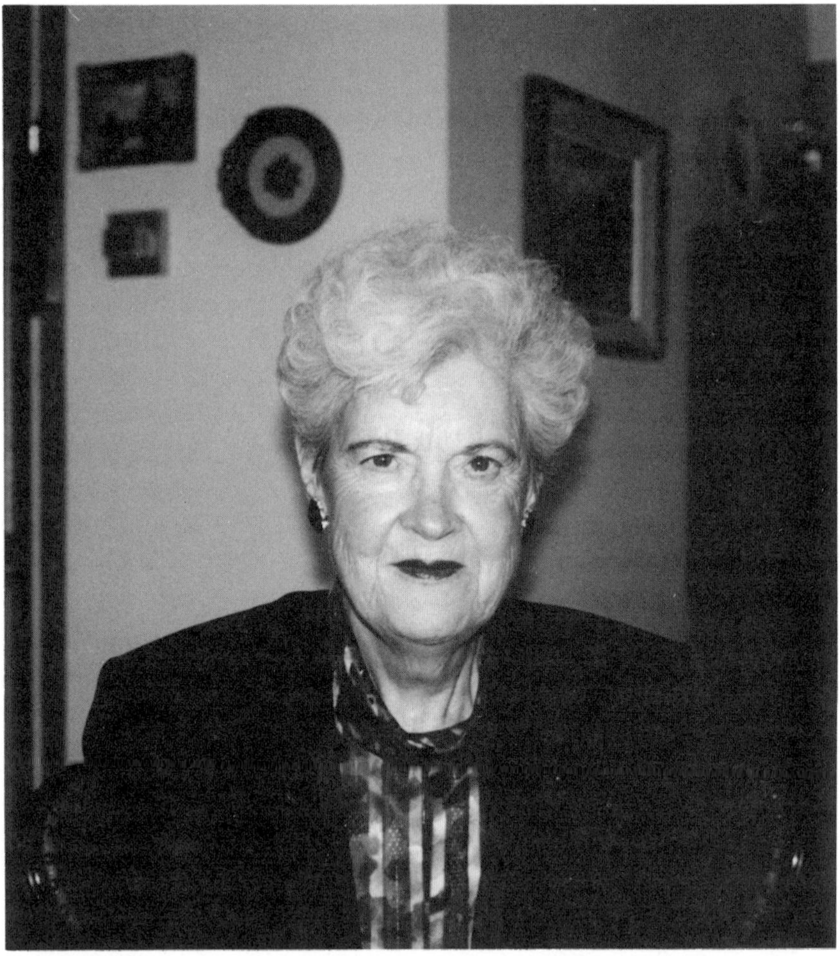

Lorna Whelan, Saskatoon, February 1995. Photo courtesy Miriam Clemence

— Chapter 4 —

Researching, Writing

CLINICAL research played a large role in David Baltzan's medical practice. He was known for the high quality of the records he kept of patient histories, and, like any serious researcher, he accepted the responsibility for the sharing of his findings. Copies of his papers appearing in the *Canadian Medical Association Journal* dating back to 1933 would make a book in themselves.

Heart and respiratory diseases were Baltzan's special field and were the subjects of his most extensive papers, but referrals to his practice brought in many other unusual cases as well, which he also brought to the attention of the profession through his publications.

In May 1933 the *Journal* reproduced in its entirety a lengthy paper[1] on digitalis administration that he had presented the previous autumn at the annual meeting of the Saskatchewan Medical Association. It was early in his internal medicine practice and doubtless he was addressing many older and more experienced physicians. Nevertheless, the tone of his address rings with confidence. By then he had years of overseas study to his credit, as well as his time at Johns Hopkins.

His extensive reading and his own clinical experience had led him to certain conclusions about the drug, of which, he said at the outset, "a perfect and final knowledge has not been acquired." The search for ''purer principles or improved whole-drug preparations'' so far had not been successful. It was unfortunate that digitalis leaf was the only form of the drug to turn to. The claims and counterclaims by manufacturers for their own brands of digitalis were confusing to practitioners, and in any case their preparations were not ''pure''. Pure digoxin had not yet appeared and attempts at standardization of preparations from the foxglove leaf were unreliable. Since little else was available by way of treatment, his paper was designed to bring practitioners abreast of developments in the use of the medication.

The coverage was thorough and went into the pharmacology and use of digitalis well beyond the issue of commercial claims. He concluded with a list of seven ''don'ts''. Among these was an admonition not to use the drug as a routine preparation for surgery unless the patient suffered from congestive failure; not to use it post-operatively with anaesthesia in cases of collapse, nor in the early stages of coronary catastrophes.

It may or may not have been Baltzan's first major address to an audience of his peers, but it certainly set the standard for his communications thereafter — clear writing and reasoned positions and the patient-first courage he was known for throughout his years of practice.

* * *

David Baltzan might very well have been the first medical practitioner to wonder out loud just what role tobacco might be playing in making people sick.

In the fall of 1933, the *Journal* ran his brief submission, ''A Significant Sign in Coronary Occlusion'',[2] in which he noticed a rather curious thread running through the histories of victims of heart attack: many, previously addicted to tobacco, had lost all interest in smoking. Baltzan wrote:

> Before attaching any significance to the observation to be described, we were impressed on several occasions by patients volunteering the statement that they had no desire to smoke since the onset of their illness.

Many not only lost their taste for tobacco in the days immediately following their attacks, but they were also ''guarded'' in their return to the habit during convalescence. Baltzan took to indirectly questioning his heart attack patients about smoking:

> This is done by approaching the subject indirectly and in such a manner as to elicit a voluntary expression. No attempt is made to imply in the interrogation the answer we anticipate.

He took pains to qualify his observations and not to attach too great a significance to the tobacco connection:

> We would be reluctant in an obscure case to accept the diagnosis without further reserve.

The clinical research he reported in the article convinced him the connection went beyond the obscure, however. He cited three cases of heart disease in which he believed smoking had been a contributory cause of the condition. From these cases he inferred that a patient's smoking history should always be determined, particularly when heart or lung disease was suspected. ''Its importance can only be established by more extensive observation,'' he wrote, concluding that he was offering his observations in the hope of ''exciting comment.'' We can only speculate what must have gone through his mind in later years as the ''comment'' he hoped for became a barrage linking tobacco use with disease.

A year later, Baltzan was back at the lectern speaking to the Moose Jaw Medical Society on ''The Management of the Cardiac Case''.[3] He began by defining the cardiac case as ''a therapeutic enigma,'' and suggesting that a large percentage of sufferers were either ''too energetically treated or sadly under treated.''

He split his paper into three parts: acute, chronic and potential, and presented state-of-the-art information in each part. It may not have been especially noticeable to his audience that day, but Baltzan was beginning to turn his attention, under the ''potential'' category, to prevention of heart disease. It was an issue, like tobacco use, that he was addressing well ahead of most in the profession. The *Journal* published his paper the following September.

In 1936, the sad case of a 15-year-old victim of Wilson's disease was presented in a Baltzan paper entitled ''Hepato-Cerebral Syndrome'':

> The interest in this case centres on the calcium deficiency factor, the extensive naked-eye pathological cerebral changes, and because in other ways it conforms to a known group entity of certain brain changes with extensive liver cirrhosis. In the Hösslin and Alzheimer pseudo-sclerosis, the pathological changes are not visible to the naked eye and are diffusely scattered throughout the greater part of the brain. The changes in Wilson's disease are macroscopic, but confined to the putamen of the lenticular nucleus. The consensus favours the view that pseudosclerosis and progressive lenticular nucleus degeneration are essentially the same disease.[4]

He then described in detail the case of the youth, who had been admitted to St. Paul's Hospital in 1933 with loss of control of his limbs, pronounced on the right side, and stiffness in his legs:

> It was obvious that there was a spastic condition of the extremities and marked disability due to incoordination in performing finer movements, and an irritability of muscle groups was noted in the course of manipulation.

After several more periods of hospitalization and extensive testing, a diagnosis of chronic tetany was made and of probable progressive lenticular degeneration of Wilson:

> A variation of the syndrome of Wilson was also postulated, having in mind a parathyroid analogue of the hepatic involvement in this disease. Positive hepatic failure could not be demonstrated at any time during the illness.

The patient died in 1935 from, according to the autopsy, "bilateral cerebral softening (encephalomalacia); chronic hepatitis; myocardial degeneration."

In 1937 Baltzan had papers published on pituitary cachexia,[5] and on experiences in Saskatchewan with 57 brucellosis infections,[6] known as the common "undulant fever," a condition transmitted to humans through infected milk in the days when pasteurization was not compulsory. The disease in cattle, called "bangs" by farmers and ranchers, led to abortion of calves. Among rural dwellers it was common to drink raw unpasteurized milk, and as Baltzan's clinical research revealed, brucellosis, or undulant fever, was prevalent at the time. A large majority of the cases he reported were chronic, with little or no consequences for the patient except in conjunction with other conditions or circumstances, such as overwork or the onset of "flu."

One of the 57 had died, though the cause of death was attributed in the main to pre-existing disease. In acute cases, Baltzan concluded, the brucellosis was "always the primary disabling factor":

> The chronic infections are by far the commonest and the diagnosis is even more elusive. Clinical groups are cited which seem to show a special predilection for occurrence of the infection. This knowledge serves as a clue to the more frequent discovery of the offending condition.

The brucellosis problem had by then attracted the attention of the province's ministry of health, which had declared the disease in cattle to be reportable.

Also in 1937, Baltzan presented "Diagnosis of Some Major Vascular Accidents"[7] at the annual meeting of the Canadian Medical Association. In the paper, published the following January in the *Journal,* he returned to a theme touched on five years earlier:

> A further (diagnostic) aid . . . is noted in those who smoke. When an occlusive process developed, it is observed that there is a loss of taste for tobacco, and the smoker automatically breaks with the habit, either permanently or until he is well on to recovery.

In 1939, the April edition of the *Journal* carried a Baltzan submission entitled "The Treatment of Angina Pectoris".[8] It emphasized the importance of an accurate diagnosis at the onset of the pain, and described the latest techniques for identifying its source and for determining its severity.

In September 1940 he wrote about a lesser known medical problem in an article entitled "Bronchomoniliasis in Saskatchewan."[9]:

> As a result of stubbornly pursuing what seemed to be an elusive cause of the disease in two persons with unusual lung manifestations, I am able to report finding bronchomoniliasis in Saskatchewan.

He gave extensive accounts of the two cases. Both resembled the debilitation of tuberculosis, but in spite of countless sputum examinations the specimens were always negative for TB. The sufferers were reduced to a severe state of disability. None of the conventional non-specific treatments helped. Baltzan finally gave deep X-ray therapy to the chests of both patients. One recovered quickly. The second had an up and down recovery, returning to normal after about six months. Baltzan did not report the radiation doses given.

> We used iodides . . . without results, perhaps because our doses were too small. We did, however, find deep X-ray therapy exceedingly beneficial.

Whether the therapy itself had any future consequences is not known. Changes in standards concerning the use of radiotherapy over the years bring questions to mind that no one would have even begun to consider at that time.

Baltzan was trying with his paper to alert others to the difficulties of diagnosing the rare disease:

> The diagnosis of bronchomoniliasis cannot be made at the bedside. The lessons . . . are: (1) to find the fungus or yeast-like cells; (2) to identify the fungus by culture; (3) to respect evidence of any wandering pneumonitis beginning with a hilar fan, which is demonstrated best by repeated roentgenograms; (4) to pay attention to the complaint of any yeast-like taste or beer-like fermentation of the sputum; (5) to bear in mind the diagnosis because it is probably more common than hereto found.

In September 1944, Baltzan was back before an audience of his peers, this time in Saskatoon at the annual meeting of the Saskatchewan Division of the Canadian Medical Association. The CMA *Journal* carried his paper in full the following August.[10] In ''Procedure in the Treatment of Heart Disease'', Baltzan devoted a section to the prevention theme:

> Cure in heart disease is minimal. The best achievement is patchwork, which is not a negligible accomplishment. In an effort to survey the means of prevention, notice will have to be taken of

> the following: (1) Early detection of defects. (2) Accurate sifting of those masquerading as cases of heart disease. (3) Special attention and accurate classification of the youthful victims in order to direct them vocationally. (4) Shortening illness but lengthening convalescence. (5) Occupational elasticity with economic security to reallocate the incapacitated for comfort, and productiveness in other jobs, to make it possible to live with disease. (6) Accelerated research in the ravages of the deficiencies and generations, to tackle the problem of the withering processes of life. (7) Lastly, to better control vital statistics or not take them too literally. Too hurried declarations of death are not accurate criteria from which to start.

His paper is notable for at least two of the ground-breaking ideas he was introducing: the whole notion of the responsibility of employers towards their employees' health, and the idea of tackling "the withering processes of life." There is no indication as to how his address was received, but it must have stirred some concern in the hearts of those in business circles who were giving little thought to employee welfare at a time when the post-war flood of willing hands meant they could pick and choose with impunity whom they put on their payrolls.

Baltzan was involved in teaching from his early years in medical practice, and he saw a need in the 1940s for a new text for nursing schools. The result was publication in 1945 of *Principles of Internal Medicine,*[11] a 398-page hardcover volume that was used extensively and is still in university and nursing school libraries.

Then in April 1950, in the first of four of his papers that the *Journal* ran that year, he and his partner Harold Sugarman authored "Hereditary Cyanosis."[12]

The paper discussed at length the research background to the identification of a genetic abnormality that was responsible for some cases of cyanosis (blueness of the blood) previously blamed on congenital heart defects. After diagnosing a whole family some 10 years earlier as suffering from cyanosis not due to heart disease, Baltzan, in association with University of Saskatchewan president and geneticist W.P. Thompson, discovered the cause was an hereditary blood pigment, methemoglobin.

Methemoglobin cannot bind molecular oxygen and therefore cannot transport oxygen around the body. Thus, an individual with this condition whose blood contains small quantities of inherited methemoglobin has the dusky appearance of cyanosis, but is otherwise perfectly well and leads a normal life, unlike a patient with cyanosis due to heart disease, in which the cyanosis is caused by insufficient oxygen in the blood.

The discovery made medical history and Baltzan was asked to name the new haemoglobin that was formed by the structural abnormality. He eschewed the personal honour and chose haemoglobin Saskatoon, symbolized by the formula HgbMs, as opposed to HgbMb.

Baltzan was quoted several years later as ruefully observing of this gesture, ''There was no ripoff from the city council for this additional honour to the City of Saskatoon, probably because it might compete with the berry — *per contra* it may be complementary.''

In May 1950, ''The Present Status of the Medical Treatment of Hypothyroidism'', appeared in the *Journal*.[13] It was a paper he had written at the request of the editors.

Another joint Baltzan/Sugarman article, ''Primary Splenic Neutroprenia with Rheumatoid Arthritis'' appeared in July,[14] followed in September by ''Uncontrollable Hives'',[15] a study of a rare condition written by Baltzan on his own.

In 1955, he expanded on his earlier beliefs on coronary disease in a paper entitled ''Anginal Syndromes''.[16]

A few years later, Baltzan was swept up in one of the most compelling issues of the times, the creation of a health care system for the entire country. The exhausting participation in the work of the royal commission headed by his old friend, Chief Justice Emmett Hall of the Supreme Court of Canada, was his main preoccupation for the first half of the 1960s, though he did still keep up his practice.

In fact, his practice grew during this period by leaps and bounds as one by one his three sons, Marc, Donald and Richard, completed their medical training and came home to join the clinic staff.

David stayed in the forefront of both the practice and the politics of medicine. As one of a selected group of physicians across the country he was asked in 1972 by the *CMAJ* editors to comment on proposals for a Community Health Centre Project contained in a report to a national conference of provincial and federal ministers of health.

The headline over his brief response summarizes his attitude: ''An impediment to the evolutionary process.'' In the article[17], he was at his bluntest best in denouncing the community clinic idea:

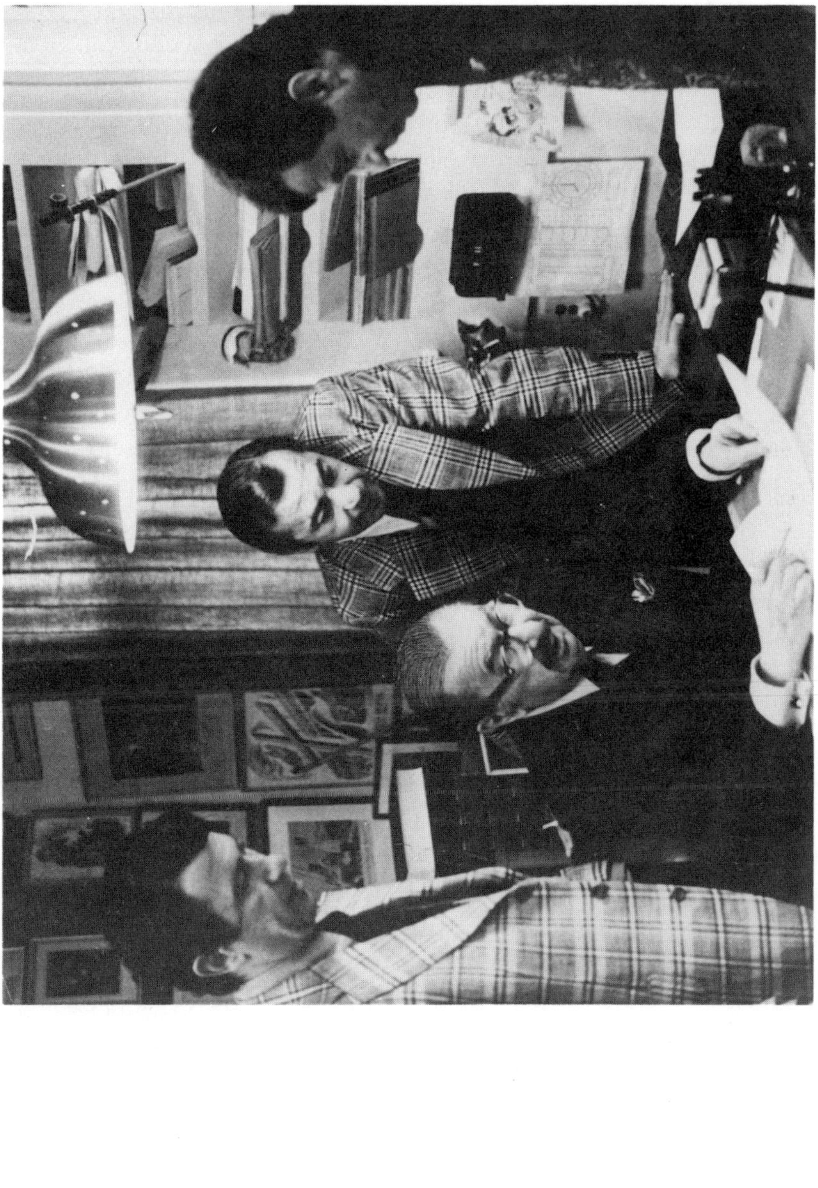

The Baltzan medical dynasty: Donald (left), David (seated), Richard and Marc

> Current community health clinics with dedicated captivated supporters have not proved what they claim — lower operational costs, increasing patronage and remedies of abuses attributed to other older systems of medical practice.
>
> There is no room to be polite confronting the proposed extravaganza . . . The already established health services are modern, convenient, and equal to the best in the world.

The heat in his response might have seemed out of character for a man whom most regarded as urbane and civil to a fault, but David Baltzan had put a great deal of himself into the system he described as "already established health services."

Part of the model was the private clinic the Baltzan family operated, a facility for decades in the forefront of diagnostic equipment and technique. Implicit in the proposals for community health clinics was the allegation that private clinics represented medicine for profit. David Baltzan and a handful of other practitioners who had given freely of their services and cancelled millions of dollars in billings in the depression years saw in private clinics a vision of service first, profits, if ever, last.

As well, of course, the national medicare system Baltzan and other members of the Hall Commission had recommended had only just been set up.

In most jurisdictions, Saskatchewan being a notable exception because it already had medicare, it meant accessible and affordable care to people who had never before known such a service. Again, the proposals for community clinics with salaried doctors flew in the face of the careful compromise the Hall Commission had devised between fee-for-service practice and state-employed doctors.

As things turned out, the community clinic model did not achieve the wide acceptance hoped for by those who made the original proposals to the health ministers. Twenty years later, most medical practices still operate along the lines of those so stoutly defended by Baltzan and others.

David Baltzan never did stop trying to improve the delivery of quality medicine on a national scale. Not long before his retirement from practice, he heralded telemetric medical services in an article in the CMA *Journal* of 3 May 1975:

> A tool of new dimensions for transmitting clinical signs of a patient instantly, either from one room to the next or thousands of miles, is now a reality.[18]

Transmissions could be auditory, pictorial, in script or hieroglyphics. Baltzan was quick to point out that this was a communications tool only, with the obvious drawback that the doctor/patient relationship would be missing from the electronic encounter. He stipulated that only doctors, trained nurses or paramedics should transmit or receive data thus exchanged.

The new system was a great breakthrough for isolated doctors who needed a second opinion or a consultation with a specialist. That was an area of personal significance to Baltzan who, as a specialist, had doubtless been asked to render opinions by telephone to outlying areas on the basis of scanty information. The telemetric system would transmit over phone lines temperature, pulse, respiration pattern, electrocardiogram, blood pressure, phenocardiogram and electroencephalogram, and other data, all of which were part of the basic information leading to a diagnosis, and all through a system of leads attached directly to the patient.

The system had been developed by Dr. M.E. Silverstein at the University of Arizona in Tucson. Baltzan had been invited there to assess the system. He was obviously pleased with what he saw and told a newspaper reporter back in Saskatoon the following month that the device would ''most definitely be adopted for the purposes of being 'a voice in the wilderness' in far-flung areas of northern Saskatchewan.''

Baltzan was 72 at the time, nearing the end of a long and distinguished career in medicine. Perhaps that was behind this philosophical passage in the *CMAJ* article:

> The spectacle of the men on the moon separated from us by a distance never travelled by human beings before, who walked in space making 'one small step for man — one giant step for mankind,' returning safely to be decontaminated from heavenly particles before joining the earthly human race, was sensational, no doubt, to the expert observers on the spot. This was not a man/machine performance, only in the sense that it was man and his creation that accounted for the accomplishment.

Doctors' responsibilities are enormous and, by nature, humanizing. That is sometimes lost in the face of a man/machine combination. The machine is supreme and compassionate; man is in limbo. That is an aberration.

— Chapter 5 —

First Kidney Transplant

IN NOVEMBER 1963, the seven-month-old Liberal minority government led by Lester Pearson was finding its way in Ottawa. The capital city was still reeling from the plots and subplots of the last days of the discredited Diefenbaker Conservatives. A few hundred miles to the south, President John F. Kennedy fell to an assassin's bullet in Dallas, Texas. A shaken American public and a shocked world struggled to cope with the sudden demise of the Camelot that had been the 35th presidency.

On the scientific front, the post-war leap into the nuclear age made all things seem possible: manned space travel; a TV revolution in communication; computers; a man on the moon? Just give us a few years.

New ways were being found to treat old diseases. Medical science was on the threshold of a golden age of unprecedented technological growth and change. Nevertheless, even though human ingenuity was soaring to new heights in research laboratories, some afflictions continued to impose relentless death sentences, among them kidney failure.

True, there was a new procedure available known as dialysis — at that time a rudimentary method for keeping patients alive temporarily by cleaning the blood artificially when the kidneys would no longer perform — but it was viewed with suspicion, looked on as little more than a source of false hope. The technology was still in doubt and the ethics

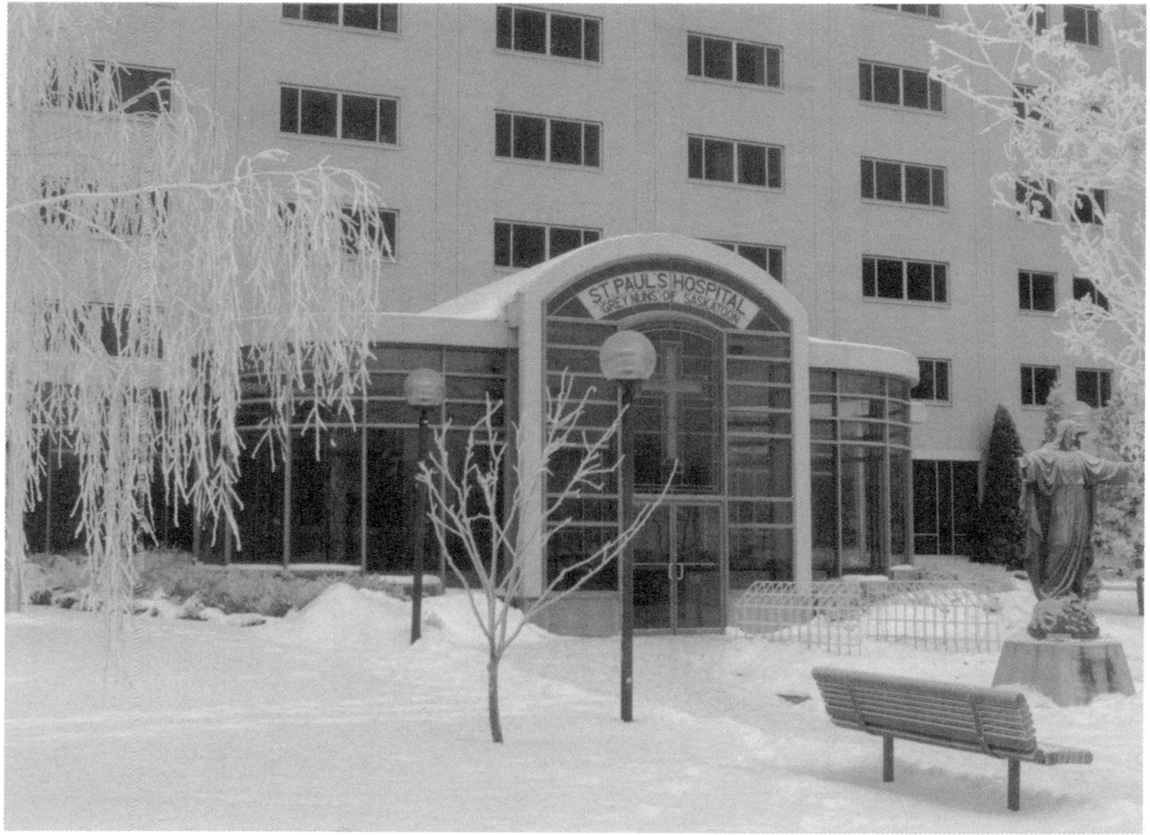

St. Paul's Hospital, Saskatoon. Photo courtesy Miriam Clemence

of the procedure were questioned by many in the medical profession and the public — though not by those whose lives it prolonged.

A handful of practitioners, however, believed in both the idea and the effectiveness of dialysis and were looking beyond to longer-term solutions for sufferers of irreversible renal failure. For certain cases, they believed kidney transplants were the answer.

By the fall of 1963, the first hesitant steps had been taken. Though fewer than 20 actual transplants had been performed around the world, and only one in Canada, the procedure was well advanced in laboratories and was beginning to attract both attention and controversy.

Public reaction to the idea of organ acquisition and transplantation ranged from one extreme to the other. Opinion was almost as sharply divided among health care professionals. The transplant question bore all the signs of a demarkation line between old-style medicine, long accustomed to simply identifying the terminal stage of mortal diseases (kidney failure among them) and making dying patients as comfortable as possible, and a new force which refused to accept that effective treatments could not be found.

Such was the backdrop to a last-ditch attempt to save the life of an 18-year-old woman with renal failure who was admitted to St. Paul's Hospital in Saskatoon under the care of the Baltzan Clinic. St. Paul's was one of three major hospitals serving a population of some 500 000 in northwest Saskatchewan and David Baltzan was its chief of medical staff.

* * *

In the autumn of 1963, the fate of the young woman had become a pressing question at the Baltzan Clinic. David's son Marc, who had followed his father's footsteps through McGill and Johns Hopkins before joining the practice in Saskatoon, and whose recollections of that baffling case were still sharp 30 years later,[1] recalled, "This woman had been perfectly well, and then one day her kidneys stopped, never to work again. It was the only thing in her body that was broken."

Most hospitals did not have dialysis machines, but the Baltzan Clinic had joined with a Saskatoon urologist to purchase one for St. Paul's.

"She came to us because she heard we had the machine. We dialysed her, but in those days it was considered immoral to try long-term dialysis . . . it was generally felt that it was absolutely certain long-term cases could not be sustained."

David, who had spent a lifetime battling diseases generally accepted as fatal, especially those affecting the heart and respiratory system, was determined to do whatever they could to help the young woman.

The question was, how to treat her?

Marc and his wife Betty Lou, a resident at University Hospital, dropped in at a party at the home of some friends one evening shortly after the woman's admission to St. Paul's. Preoccupied with the woman's condition, the two began a conversation with a urologist and other medical colleagues about the case.

''We didn't know what to do,'' Marc recalled, until the discussion turned to transplants. ''Then, somehow, it was conceived that the woman would be a good candidate for the procedure.''

In a library search, Betty Lou found reports on 15 transplants around the world, all within the previous 12 months. The use of a new drug, Azathioprine, to help the recipient of the organ fight rejection had led to the spate of operations. The Baltzans studied the data. They decided the procedure was rational and possible. Two surgeons began at once to practise transplants on dogs in the lab.

The next step was to find a donor. The idea of using newly deceased donors sharply exacerbated the ethical objections to transplants. Worse, no recipient of a kidney from a dead donor had yet lived. Only patients who had received kidneys from living donors to whom they were related had survived. The Baltzans approached the mother of the stricken 18-year-old to ask her for one of her kidneys. She agreed. The stage was set.

But the Baltzans were uneasy.

''We began to get cold feet,'' Marc said.

They sought the help of their colleagues and convened what was possibly the first ethics committee at University Hospital in Saskatoon. A representative of the hospital administration was invited, along with several doctors who were not personally involved with the case and lawyers and clerics. The discussions were intense. In the end, approval was not unanimous, but it was enough to satisfy the Baltzans that they should proceed.

Marc relates an incident that illustrates the depth of the moral and ethical soul-searching. David's friend Jim Campbell, the urologist with whom the Baltzans had jointly purchased the dialysis machine, declared that he would not involve himself in the transplant. He had decided the procedure was ethically unacceptable. He assured David that he was not trying to impose his own morality, however, and urged the team to carry on.

It was high drama. Marc oversaw the intricate preparations[2] as the ethical questions behind the decision to perform the operation continued to swirl in the hospital corridors. The team was assembled.

While David nervously waited outside, Marc observed the procedure inside the operating room. The operation was carried out by a surgeon named Neville Jackson.

''I'll never forget,'' Marc reflected, still with a note of awe in his voice. ''He put the kidney in, hooked up the blood vessels and turned the ureter up, and urine shot out six inches or a foot, instantly. I don't think I've ever been so excited in my life.''

The elated operating team stayed at the hospital late into the night — but their joy was short lived.

Shortly after arriving home about midnight, Marc's phone rang. The kidney had stopped working. Marc remembers how distraught he and his father were, and he recalls also how he and Betty Lou encountered Jim Campbell in the operating room corridor at University Hospital the next day.

Campbell, the doubter who had approached David earlier, ''put his arm around my shoulders and told me not to give up, to keep trying. That meant an awful lot.''

Two years later, David and Marc learned that the cause of the failure was hyperacute rejection, in which antibodies had lain ''in ambush'' before surgery. Today, such 'ambushes' are thwarted by pre-operative testing for incompatibility between organ and host. The reaction was not understood at the time, being the first case in North America, and only the second in the world (a similar failure was reported in Paris).

With the transplant failure, a chronic dialysis system had to be created before the remaining kidney failed completely.

''I remember we jimmied up a system . . . actually we manufactured it in the engineering lab on Christmas day that year,'' Marc said.

The idea of a second attempt at a kidney transplant had not been abandoned. Early in the new year, Marc and Betty Lou happened to be in Virginia visiting relatives when they heard of a doctor named David Hume who was performing kidney transplants at the Medical College of Virginia. Hume was from Boston, where he had worked with Joe

Murray, winner of a Nobel Prize in medicine for his work on kidney transplants of the previous year.

Hume encouraged the Baltzans. He had patients who were still living a year after having had kidney transplants. Some of those operations had been performed using cadaver organs. Back in Saskatoon, the Baltzans got a phone call on 22 February to say a brain-dead donor was available. Marc remembers what happened next.

"We looked at each other, and we said, 'Well, if it is, it is,' and we went ahead and got consent and we did it (the second transplant)."

The procedure was a success and the woman lived for four months. She died after contracting hepatitis when she moved to a mining camp in pursuit of her husband, who had deserted her.

The true significance of that first transplant at University Hospital — now Royal University Hospital — in Saskatoon wasn't recognized at first. The controversy around the ethics of transplants in general continued. The public was only marginally aware in the early 1960s of the issues involved in kidney transplantation, and of course had no idea of the wide range of other medical science sagas to come.

Once the transplant genie was out of the bottle, however, there was no stopping it. Within a comparatively short period the procedure was treated as routine at the Saskatoon hospital and elsewhere. In the 30 years following that first Canadian transplant engineered by the Baltzans, an estimated 565 patients in Saskatchewan alone have received kidneys and new leases on life. Across Canada, an estimated 2100 people were on waiting lists in late 1993, including 70 in Saskatchewan. The operation itself has been refined over the years and new and better drugs have been developed to combat rejection which, with the shortage of donors, still haunts transplant programs everywhere.

The roles played by the Baltzans and Saskatoon's University Hospital has kept both in the forefront of kidney transplantation. Seven of the 33 longest-living recipients of cadaveric kidney transplants are from Saskatoon.[3] Seventy-eight per cent of patients in the province who received kidneys from live donors have lived for 18 years or more, the highest rate recorded.

That first transplant and the accompanying soul-searching for many doctors in Saskatoon are both indicative of the role played by David Baltzan, both in his own practice and in the medical community as a whole. His views were respected. The support he provided typified the relationships among the partners in the Baltzan Clinic over their years of working together. The younger members always knew David was in charge, yet he did not interfere. Differences in knowledge and attitude worked themselves out. What evolved was a combination of a ''young man's'' and an ''old man's'' medicine,[4] the young representing ''body mechanics,'' or using what you learn in medical school, the old the judgment side, the part that comes from knowing and understanding people.

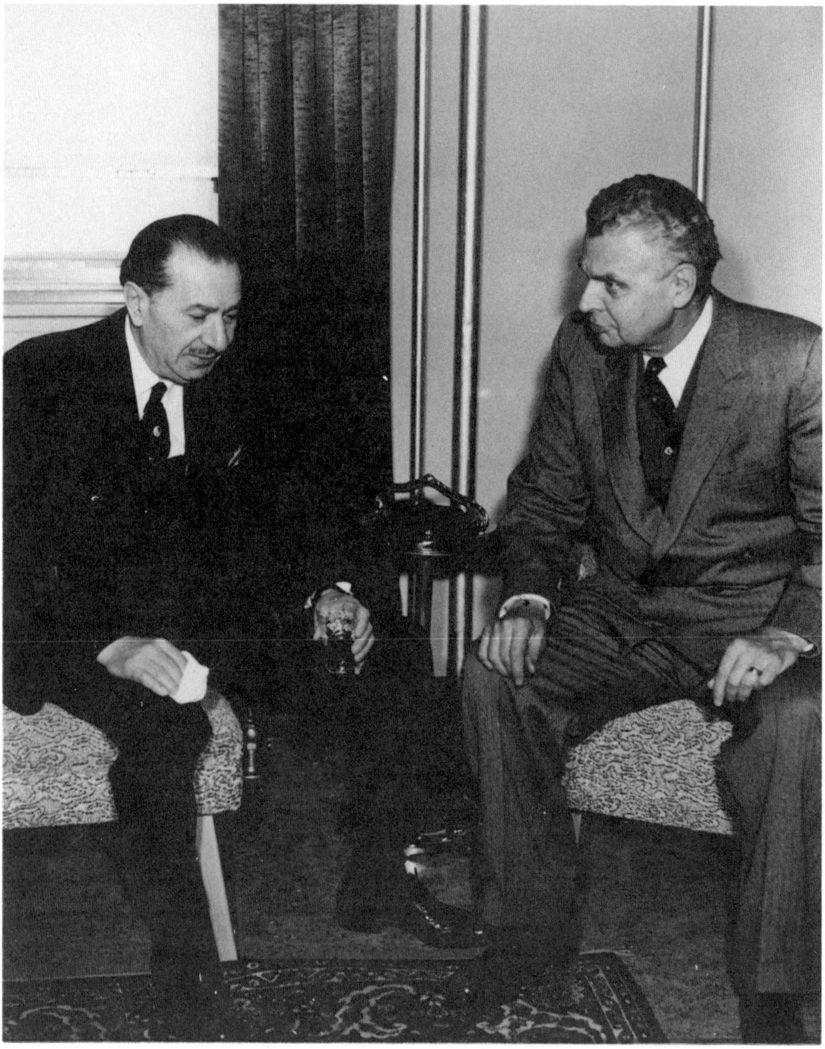

David Baltzan in conversation with his longtime friend John Diefenbaker

Chapter 6
Pen Pal Dief

DAVID BALTZAN could best be described as a "people" person, as distinct from an individual with pronounced political ambition or entrepreneurial passions. He made no bones about his life-long political loyalties, however. He was a Progressive Conservative supporter, and sometimes even indulged in the political rhetoric of the day. But he was not a doctrinaire rightist, and today's neo-conservatives in Canada would in all likelihood be hard put to recognize him as one of their own from his pragmatic philosophy.

Marc, in fact, doubts his father actually had a political philosophy. He speculates that David became a Conservative back in the 1920s when every other immigrant was a member of the Liberal party. "I think there was streak of contrariness in my father. And I think what he really desired was to be part of the country where he lived, and not to maintain an individual, ritualistic orientation."

In a state of political ambivalence or not, Baltzan was comfortably attuned to the thinking of his long-time friend, John George Diefenbaker. Dief the Chief, as the legendary politician was fondly known in his home province, has been described as an "eloquent spokesman for nonestablishment Canada," both in his tempestuous law practice, when he defended unpopular individuals and unpopular causes alike, and when he was prime minister in later life.

Baltzan and Diefenbaker, with their friend Emmett Hall, were the reddest of red Tories in the view of some of their less supportive eastern counterparts. But if their brand of politics frightened the party establishment, it certainly had no such effect on the country as a whole. Diefenbaker, with piercing gaze and thundering oratory, swept out of political obscurity in the West. The charismatic lawyer imbued his listeners with his eloquent vision of a youthful Canada coming into its own as an egalitarian, caring society rich in resources, particularly of the human variety.

Diefenbaker, in fact, was a towering figure on the national scene for close to a decade. Born in Ontario in 1895, he moved with his family to the Fort Carlton area of the Northwest Territories in 1903. His education at the University of Saskatchewan was interrupted by the Great War. When he returned from overseas service, he completed his schooling and was called to the bar in Saskatchewan in 1919. After operating a one man practice at Wakaw for a time, he moved to Prince Albert in 1924.

Then, while David Baltzan was defying conventional wisdom by building up a practice in the unpromising specialty of internal medicine in Saskatoon, Diefenbaker began to march to the beat of a different drummer altogether. Political ambition and a reformer's zeal had driven him from an early age. Seeing political office as the route to bringing about change, he ran for a federal seat in 1925 and 1926, then for the provincial legislature in 1929, the mayoralty of Prince Albert in 1933, and the legislature again in 1938.

The voters rejected him every time.

Eventually he succeeded in winning the leadership of the provincial Conservative party in 1936, but again tasted failure when the party was unable to win even one seat in the Saskatchewan election of 1938.

Diefenbaker was nothing if not persistent. His persistence finally paid off when he was elected to the House of Commons in 1940 as a Conservative MP for the Saskatchewan riding of Lake Centre in Regina. He won the seat twice more, in 1945 and 1949, sitting as a member of the opposition until redistribution did away with the riding.

Diefenbaker decided to get out of politics, but within a few years, local supporters convinced him to stand for nomination again on his home turf in Prince Albert. These supporters were a loose collection of bipartisan individuals who called themselves the "Diefenbaker Club".[1] Among their numbers were many Liberals and card-carrying NDPers as well as Tories and people with no political ties whatsoever, united in one thing only — their admiration for Dief and his vaunted political skills.

Ever the outlaw, Diefenbaker would not allow a Progressive Conservative party banner in his campaign headquarters (except for TV cameras), and he battled the national party executive even as prime minister and its leader. He won the election and was back in the House in 1953 where his fortunes continued to rise. He was a surprise winner in the federal Progressive Conservative leadership race of 1956, following the resignation of George Drew. In 1957, Diefenbaker and the Progressive Conservatives defeated the Liberals and their failing leader Louis St. Laurent, taking over the reigns of government by a narrow margin. The gain was consolidated in 1958 when The Chief led his party to the largest Conservative victory to that date with 208 seats.

His glory days were short-lived, however. Though he made a name for himself and the country among Commonwealth nations as a friend and supporter, opened up markets for western wheat in communist countries, enacted his own Bill of Rights and set the process in motion that eventually led to Medicare in Canada, a domestic economic crisis dimmed his hopes for a strong second term.

In 1962, the PCs barely won enough votes to form a minority government against the Liberals and their new leader Lester Pearson. When they went back to the people the following year, hoping for a renewed majority, the Pearson Liberals came out on top.

Diefenbaker's political battles were not over, however. As it turned out, his worst enemies were in his own party. In a bitterly fought leadership campaign in 1967, he lost out to Robert Stanfield. The distinctive Diefenbaker style was muted on Parliament Hill, though the once-revered figure still occupied a seat near the front of the opposition benches, from which he could be heard day after day pounding the government and his arch-rival Pearson.

Prince Albert voters sent The Chief back for 13 more years, his last election victory coming in 1979, the year of his death.

Among the stacks of papers he left behind, which were still being sorted and filed at the Diefenbaker Centre on the University of Saskatchewan campus in Saskatoon 15 years after his death, are scores of the letters he and David Baltzan exchanged over the years to keep their association strong.

Baltzan provided many services for his old friend, both of a personal and a political nature. One of the most important topics of their written exchanges was the health of Diefenbaker's mother. Mother and son were very close and Baltzan was in charge of Mrs. Diefenbaker's care when she fell seriously ill in 1957. While Diefenbaker's political career was taking off, Baltzan was sending him frequent updates, such as this one dated the 4th of November:

> I enclose again a duplicate of the hospital chart which describes the 'spells.' I regret I cannot withhold the information as I have done so many times in the past when it was clinically safe for me to do so . . . I will only write or call you when things look clearly better or worse.

The chart reports that the patient was "hostile toward staff, eyes very reddened . . . disoriented as to time and place . . . argumentative . . ."

Diefenbaker's belated reply came from Nassau, Bahamas, on December 29, obviously after he had received more reports on his mother's condition, perhaps by phone or via the telegrams he and Baltzan often exchanged:

> . . . I am indebted to you for everything you have done for mother, and while a message by letter cannot convey my feelings as could be achieved by a personal chat, I want you to know that I am grateful to you.

Baltzan lost his own mother the following February, which brought a note of condolence from the Prime Minister. Then in early April a letter arrived from Diefenbaker in Bermuda. He apologized for failing to get in touch with Baltzan during a recent stopover in Saskatoon and again conveyed "deep regard and appreciation for the exceptional care and attention you have given my mother."

On the 3rd of June that year, Baltzan wrote to report Diefenbaker's mother, still hospitalized, was better:

> Today, the physical condition is good, the attitude agreeable. The wish to go home is strong, but we all know she gets the best attention this way.

On the road again in November 1958, Diefenbaker wrote to Baltzan from a plane. The PM had visited several communist countries and was en route to Malaya, Singapore, Australia and New Zealand:

> It has been a most revealing trip and has led me to question whether the policies that the free world is following will have any appreciable effect in stemming Communism.

That was a theme the two returned to more than once. Baltzan followed Diefenbaker's activities from afar, occasionally cheering him on by telegram. After watching a Diefenbaker television performance on 20 April 1959, for example, Baltzan dashed off this telegram assessment:

> TV DELIVERY SPIRITED AND SINCERE STOP COVERAGE COMPACT AND COMPREHENSIVE STOP STATISTICS SYMBOLICALLY EFFECTIVE AND GOOD FOR EMPHASIS STOP WILL PHONE TOMORROW

The two exchanged books of common interest and often commented on their impressions of the various titles. On 19 June 1959, Baltzan began a letter to Diefenbaker on just such a note before congratulating his friend on a recent honour:

> Your views of Hover's *Life of Woodrow Wilson* affirm the impressions I derived from the book. I am pleased about your recognition by Princeton University. No honour is greater in my estimation, than the honour conferred and the trust placed on one by the great majority of one's own fellow Canadians. How to prove that worth and show my gratitude would torment me. I am doubly glad you are the Prime Minister of Canada.

Baltzan also mentioned a quandary he was in. He was scheduled to attend a medical conference in Edinburgh, Scotland, the following month—just when the Queen would be touring Canada. Although Diefenbaker's mother was a lot better, he feared the excitement of the royal visit might bring on a relapse while Diefenbaker was preoccupied with duties as head of state:

> This is what I plan: to hold on to my reservations and act according to indications with the best interests of the local position predominant. If I do not leave, it will be on account of extra precautions.

Diefenbaker's reply, marked "personal," was dated four days later:

> My Dear Doctor: Thank you for your letter . . . I see no reason whatever for you to sacrifice your trip . . . I have deputized various Ministers to accompany Her Majesty . . .I would feel very happy if you were to advise that you reconsidered the matter and decided to go on your trip.

So it was arranged, and apparently with no ill effects. By late July, with the Queen's Dominion Day (as it was then still known) tour behind him, Diefenbaker was onto another topic, beginning his letter with an observation that spoke volumes about Baltzan's value as his ears and eyes in Saskatchewan:

> Dear Doctor:
> The title that you ascribe to yourself as unofficial Minister of Local Affairs without Portfolio does not do justice to the position that you have occupied for so long. Indeed, without your constant help and kindness, things would have been almost impossible.
>
> Now for another title. As you know, the gift for Her Majesty consists of setting up a million dollar trust fund for research into children's diseases, with the fund to be administered by a Board of Directors. While it is entirely an honorary position, I wonder whether you would consider being included as one of the members.
>
> Last week I spoke at the opening ceremonies of the World Paediatrics Congress and dealt in general with the degree to which medical science crossed the ideological boundaries which separate the world. While there was nothing novel in what I stated, the views that you and I have expressed on occasion were embodied in my remarks.

Baltzan replied at once, adding a touch of humour:

> My answer is, yes, very willingly and HAZEN can't ARGUE on this point.

He was referring, of course, to Saskatchewan CCF MP Hazen Argue, the only non-Conservative to survive the Diefenbaker sweep of the province in 1958. Argue was house leader of the eight-member CCF (Co-operative Commonwealth Federation) caucus at the time and as such was a well known thorn in the side of Diefenbaker. A year later he was elected federal CCF leader. He resigned from the Federation after it became the NDP (New Democratic Party) in 1961, and ran as a Liberal in 1962. He won that election, but was defeated in 1963. He was later appointed to the Senate.

Life wasn't all honorary positions and fraternal greetings, however. In March 1960, Baltzan reported to the Prime Minister on a matter of greater substance:

> The Event in Regina was a success: we got the go-ahead sign, & it is not contingent on any Federal/Provincial arrangements, come what may. The argument about the lack of interest shown on the part of seven other provinces stuck! Our own facts and figures were not brushed aside as on previous occasions.
>
> Monteith [Hon. Waldo Monteith] gave me a trump card and I told him at the time I would not use it unless the chips were down. I didn't & spared the federal government being drawn into the crisis (for us).
>
> My visit to Ottawa was too short, too rushed & I was too moody about the coming Sunday Event. Had to prepare my strategy on the return flight to Regina. It was not a one man show, but not many could be allowed to take part.
>
> Premier D [Tommy Douglas, CCF] & I remain very good friends in spite of the tough bargaining. He has goodness in his heart, but his heart-strings got him tangled up. Erb [Saskatchewan Health Minister Walter Erb] was silent and I was glad.
>
> We are both converts — she believes in my God and I believe in her God; I am happy always to see you both — but don't ever let me become a nuisance when you have so much to do.
>
> Your Mother is in fine shape. It is a pleasure and satisfaction to see her content. Elmer [Diefenbaker's brother] is in town all this week & he will be with us Fri. & Sat.

The news was not so good by year's end. Early in December 1960, Baltzan sent copies of his clinical notes on the elderly Mrs. Diefenbaker's condition to a worried prime minister. The last line read, "remains on critical list."

> For your peace of mind, I want to restate some of my beliefs. Both in general and in the particular, I stress that I refuse to 'torture' to keep alive the 'unremedial.' On the other hand, I do everything to make 'living' easier while there is life. When there is hope for 'restoration,' everything must be done to prolong life.

The prime minister's mother passed away soon after. On 25 February 1961, Diefenbaker wrote:

> Your help and devotion to my Mother's comfort and welfare for so many years was such that no words would be adequate. What you have done will never be forgotten by Elmer and me.

But life went on:

> I was very interested in your letter dealing with the Health Committee in which you dealt with the impatience of the Chairman over some delay in the arrival of the representatives of the medical societies.

Fifteen months later, a new concern could be discerned in the correspondence. After one term with an all-powerful majority in the House, the Diefenbaker Conservatives had been reduced to minority government. On 27 June 1962, Baltzan bolstered The Chief's spirits:

> The day following the election, I tried to reach John Fisher or you, and you had just left the Air Port. I wanted to tell you, your immediate post election pronouncement was exactly what I wanted to hear. It was a perfect helmsman's stand.
>
> Emmett [Hall] told me he will see you next week. There is merit in some things he will tell you . . . As always I have complete trust that you will lead this nation out of the ravages upon its reputation by Her Majesty's (dis)-loyal opposition in and out of Parliament.

Baltzan kept close watch over Diefenbaker's political fortunes and wasn't averse to taking a hand himself when he thought his intervention might help. Such was the case when he took two national television reporters to task for their treatment of a federal Tory cabinet minister in a program he had watched. In a lengthy letter to Diefenbaker dated 15 November 1962, he mentioned the response:

> Today I received from Hon. H. Green a letter of appreciation for the telegram to Norman Depoe and Charles Lynch deploring their injudicious interrogation of the Hon. Minister on their TV interview Oct. 24th last. It was especially appreciated by him because he wrote, 'Several people have been very critical of my part' . . .

With that letter, Baltzan enclosed a clipping from *The Jewish Post* 8 November 1962:

> Ron Goldberg, son of Mrs. Anne Goldberg and the late William Goldberg, has been chosen as the first recipient of the Mr. and Mrs. M.A. Baltzan Sr. Memorial Bursary. The $500 bursary, awarded for the first time this year, is being given to a deserving university student who has graduated from the Edmonton Talmud Torah Hebrew School. The award is presented by Mrs. Marvin Dower and Ronald M. Baltzan of Edmonton, and Dr. Marcel, Dr. Richard and Dr. Donald Baltzan, all of Saskatoon, in memory of their late grandparents.

"I enclose this clipping because it pleases me so much," wrote Baltzan, ever the firm believer in education. It was an especially fitting tribute to his parents. Perhaps as he penned the observation, David was remembering his scholarly father Moishe, who set up a study centre in the milking shed on his Lipton homestead in the early 1900s so that no minds would go to waste.

By 1964, Diefenbaker was back on the opposition benches, though still immersed in measures he had initiated while he was Prime Minister, such as the Royal Commission on Health Care headed by Emmett Hall, with Baltzan as a member.

In a note to Baltzan on 23 June 1964, he commented:

> The reception regarding the Royal Commission report has been very interesting. I have scanned through it and must say I am very impressed. The style and wording of the report are quite literary.

As both men slowed the pace of their lives, Baltzan looking to retirement, Diefenbaker's star fading in the party while he became less and less active in House debates, their exchanges tended to dwell more on more personal things, though they remained interested in the affairs of the nation and continued to exchange views periodically. In November 1965, Diefenbaker dispatched a letter in which he gleefully indulged in some witty Liberal-bashing:

> I am now on my way to Ottawa, where surprising events are taking place. The resignation of the Minister of Finance (Walter Gordon) because he gave bad advice would be understandable had he belonged to the Presidium, but if British Parliamentary practice were followed, the Prime Minister and Government, and not the Minister, would resign. It seems to me that the ancient tribute to one who gives his life for his friend will now have to be altered to read: 'Greater love hath no man than this, that he lay down his friend's life for his own.'

Again, in June 1966 an indignant Diefenbaker got off some shots over the scandal involving call girl Gerda Munsinger and several cabinet ministers from the Conservative era:

> Commissioner Spence has advised me of allegations of misconduct in the Munsinger case and has asked for my explanation and I am not even going to reply, for his conclusions were formed even before the Commission actually commenced to take evidence.
>
> Mr. Fulton did not consult with me as to the course he took by way of reply to certain allegations against him. However, in today's *Globe & Mail*, a full report appears, and I am sending you the tear sheet. I have spoken to several judges about the manner in which the Commissioner conducted the proceedings of the Commission, and without exception each and every one

of them have expressed the view that the Commissioner's conduct has been appalling, and in his disregard of ordinary rules of evidence he has brought no honour to the bench.

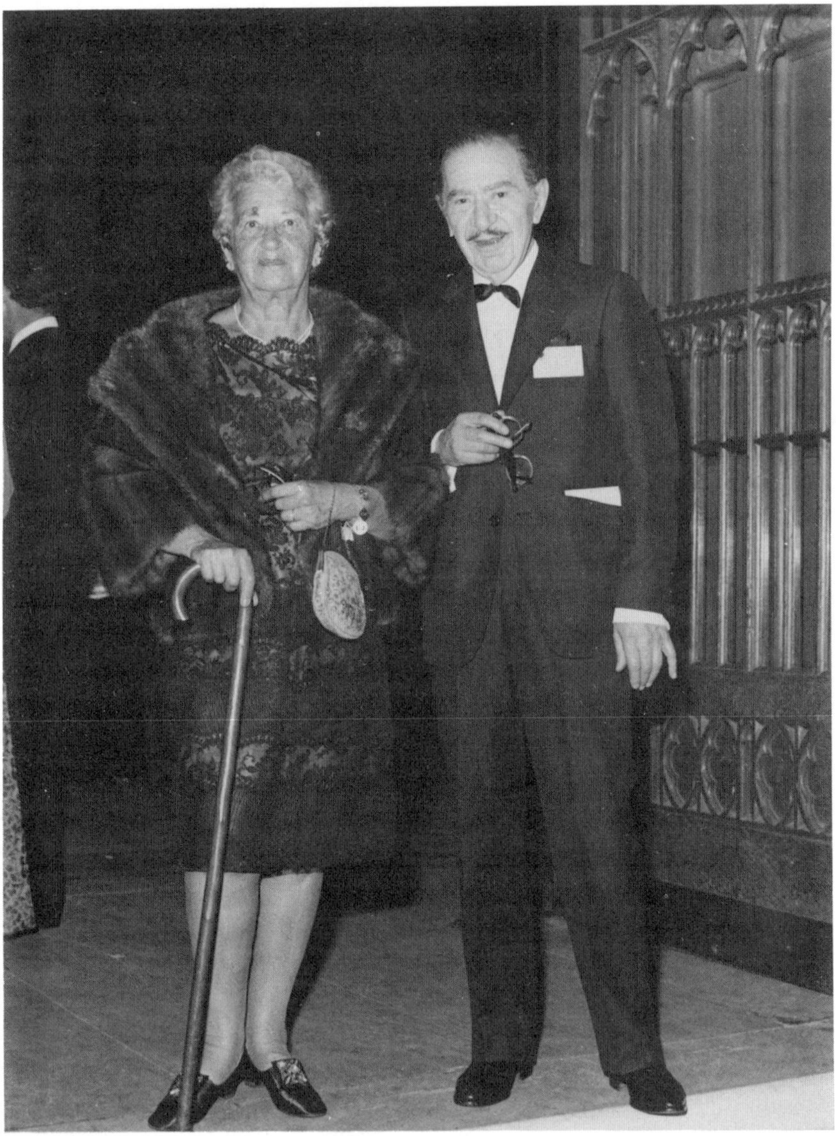

David and Rose Baltzan in London, England, in 1970 for the International Congress of Cardiologists

— Chapter 7 —

Travels Abroad

WHEN JOHN Diefenbaker invited David Baltzan in 1959 to serve on the board of trustees for the Queen Elizabeth II Canadian Fund to Aid in the Research of the Diseases of Children, he requested a list of the professional and academic posts Baltzan held at the time. The doctor complied with three single-spaced, typewritten pages of information.

The listing demonstrated the extent of Baltzan's involvement in the city and provincial medical communities. By then he had been chief of staff at St. Paul's Hospital for five years, where he had also served for 25 years as chief of the medical staff; he was associate professor of clinical medicine at the University of Saskatchewan; and he headed the educational committee of the Saskatchewan College of Physicians and Surgeons, a job he applied himself to with such zeal as to occasionally raise the ire of hard-pressed peers who had trouble finding the time to participate.

Baltzan subscribed to medical publications from near and far and read copiously to keep up with the changing scene. He was known as a thorough teacher and took an active interest in all facets of training programs for both doctors and nurses. Among the Baltzan family endowments was the Medical Canadiana Library at the University of Saskatchewan and a scholarship at a Hebrew University in Jerusalem.

Baltzan's work with heart disease extended to involvement with both provincial and national boards of the Canadian Heart Foundation. He also found time to work with both provincial and national executives of the John Howard Society and was outspoken in his support for the rights of men and women in prison. And though his involvement with the Saskatoon Jewish community was waning by 1959, he kept up his work with national and international groups. Among other activities and memberships, he served as national director of the Council of Christians and Jews and past president of B'nai B'rith Canada.

His interests in medicine, world Jewry and education took him around the world to conferences and organizational gatherings, or just on visits to learn the ways of other people. It was a matter of considerable pride to him that by 1959 he had visited every continent except Australia.

Baltzan's world vision was kindled at an early age by his own immigrant status. Later, his studies took him as a young man to Edinburgh, Vienna and the New England States for postgraduate work after attending medical school at McGill. By the time he settled down in Saskatoon to practise as an internist, he had already been exposed to all the contrasts of the old world and the new. It is hardly surprising that seeking knowledge and understanding in far-flung, disparate cultures became a lifelong pursuit.

It was just such a pursuit that took him in 1958 on a solitary odyssey through the Orient that lasted over a month and covered 22 000 air miles. A lengthy and detailed newspaper account[1] reported that Baltzan had visited Japan, Formosa (Taiwan), Thailand, Singapore and Hong Kong. He made the trip, he told reporters, because that part of the world was the focal point of global interest. Baltzan barely touched base with diplomats, either Canadian or nationals, in the places he visited, preferring, he said, to "rub shoulders" with everyday people whenever he could.

A chance conversation with some Japanese people who sat next to him at the National Theatre in Tokyo, for example, resulted in a two-day stay in a private home. On another occasion, he engaged a driver in Formosa and visited rice farms, where he talked to the farmers with the assistance of his driver, who doubled as interpreter.

Singapore was unbearably hot, busy and orderly, the city's business section as modern as any western hub of commerce. Parks and residential sections were well groomed — all, Baltzan observed, bearing testimony to the British influence upon the locals, who were nevertheless clearly in charge.

In Hong Kong he encountered evidence of the changes that were taking place in China. Refugees who sought safety in the teeming city were no fans of the Chiang Kai-shek regime, but were not enamoured of communism either. Still, the complexities of nationalism were revealed in the rejection of western ways by the Chinese. Baltzan told the Saskatoon reporters that the Chinese were "furiously fond" of their homeland.

It was not safe for Baltzan to travel overland to Thailand because of the French Indo-Chinese war, but the combatants allowed air traffic over a prescribed route on certain days. He flew right over the battlefields to get to Bangkok where, again, he shunned what he called "the board of trade angle" in favour of contact with ordinary citizens.

Japan was the country that captured most of his interest. He reported that though the scars of World War II were still relatively fresh, there was no talk of either war or peace. He was amazed to see the extent of the rebuilding going on in the cities. Everyone was engaged in reshaping the economy and culture.

He walked the streets of Hiroshima and saw The Peace Monument, the untouched city centre left as a memorial to the dead and dying from the world's first atomic bombing of a populated area. Not surprisingly, he made a point of observing the medical treatment of the various maladies that were showing up as a result of exposure to the radiation.

Baltzan concluded that the people of Japan were "making a virtue out of defeat," an attitude all the more admirable in light of the enormous scale of the war damage. He said the devastation in the country was far greater than he had expected outside Hiroshima and Nagasaki. More 'conventional' weapons had ravaged many other areas, among them the city of Tokyo, where still there were terrible slums with very poor sanitation.

Politically and socially the country had achieved a high degree of equality. After the war, Emperor worship was practised in the main only by older citizens. An example of the egalitarian measures Baltzan observed and commented upon was the uniforms worn by all school children, rich and poor alike. He noted, though, that there was still a large gender bias in and out of the family, with the status of men far superior to that of women.

Baltzan did not limit his observations to things medical when he travelled.

On one trip he made an exhaustive study of education systems under communist regimes. Back in Canada, he wrote a lengthy report for a radio broadcast and for newspapers, pointing out ways in which educational opportunities were better for children of some communist countries. He shared his findings with his old friend John Diefenbaker. In spite of the strident Cold War rhetoric of the day and the virulent anti-communism that pervaded the Western World, Diefenbaker was inclined to share Baltzan's views.

In 1956, no doubt using his connections in the External Affairs Department — he was friendly with the minister of the day, Paul Martin Sr. — Baltzan managed to get past the Iron Curtain to travel extensively through Russia to look at health care and the state of Soviet medical education. He was accompanied by Iser Steinman, another friend who practised medicine in Vancouver and who could speak fluent Russian. Baltzan could converse in several languages, Yiddish among them, but not Russian.

On his return to Canada, he prepared a detailed report, which he delivered to the annual Christmas gathering of the St. Paul's Hospital staff. It was later published in abridged form in the *Canadian Medical Association Journal*.[2]

On seeing Leningrad, Baltzan remarked how the evidence of the 900-day siege endured by its citizens during the war was still vivid. The ordeal had had many consequences for the survivors, among them a condition the Russian doctors called "blockade hypertension." They believed that months of poor nutrition and unrelieved stress had given rise to a delayed rise in blood pressure in many of the city's inhabitants.

Given the state of international tensions and the prevailing Cold War rhetoric, with Josef Stalin not long dead and Nikita Khrushchev feeling his way through hostile international waters, the Russians whom Baltzan met tended to be insular and highly suspicious of outsiders. They were doubtless surprised to find two North American doctors in their midst. Baltzan likened the welcome they received at a medical college in Leningrad to that which might have been accorded a visitor from Mars:

> I choose Mars because everywhere we went we were continually asked why we wanted war. We thought we were the least representative warlike-looking specimens in captivity.

He commented on many differences he found between the Soviet and the Canadian systems. Students in one college, for example, were trained right from the beginning of their medical courses for specific jobs, be it in public health, general practice or any other specialty.

On entrance, a student knows the end at the beginning, but the end is also the beginning of further training in the field, was how he explained it. He also found that, unlike Canadian medical schools, all Soviet medical schools operated on a uniform curriculum. He described the members of the "Cabinet of Methodology" in the Soviet Ministry of Health as "a sincere lot," though some had misgivings about the imposition of total uniformity and regimentation. He discovered that from only 16 000 students in medicine in 1913 in the Soviet Union, the number had grown to 142 000 by 1956, with about 18 000 graduating annually.

Another difference between medical education in his own country and in the Soviet system was that medical schools in the Soviet Union had been divorced from universities since 1935, when medical education was put under the control of the Ministry of Health. Baltzan was critical of the separation:

> I could not help feeling that the split would ultimately assert itself in the philosophy of medicine and the relation to its scientific application.

Of the hospitals he visited, including one in the distant republic of Uzbekistan, he wrote:

> I was favourably impressed by the physicians, surgeons and research workers and disappointed with the net results, which are not their fault. The sum total must be judged against the backdrop of the Brave New World wholesale approach to the social and economic adventure.
>
> The use of cadaver blood for blood transfusions is prevalent. The blood is removed up to six hours after death and preserved by refrigeration without citrate for three weeks. Each corpse delivers 2-4 litres of blood. Exsanguination is not made in traumatic deaths. In twenty years, 23 tons of cadaver blood was collected. It is claimed that blood transfusion reactions are reduced by 50%. Also it is a matter of necessity. Blood is otherwise hard

> to get because — it is insinuated — there is no monetary attraction to donors, and in fact, there is not the same patriotic inducement which existed during the war.

Baltzan reported that in Moscow there were eight beds per 1000 population, with an expected increase to 11-13 beds. Patient stay averaged no less than 40-45 days, "and this does not seem to trouble anybody."

He contrasted that statistic with the numbers in Canada:

> . . . We feel self-critical if the average occupation is 18-20 days and think there is laxity in the management of the patient. Free hospital care, free drugs and free medical services are not the complete solution of the problems of sickness. This is a limited view. The best treatment, the quickest cure and the surest prevention, these are the ultimates in medicine. They are not free under any system. In Russia the cost is met by individual cutbacks in the earnings of the workers because government needs so much more. The worker is paid less and charged more for the cost of living.

Baltzan was taken with one aspect of the Soviet system, however. He was intrigued by the so-called preventoriums for convalescent patients, which he allowed were "commendable adaptations to the needs for accommodation." The facilities, however, did not demonstrate any benefits of a scientific nature.

In the final analysis, he said, Soviet doctors belonged to a privileged class:

> The Soviet Union is only theoretically a classless society.

He worried over the emphasis on teamwork in Soviet medicine, saying this "collectivism" was overrated. He believed western medicine was leaning too much in the same direction:

> Self-expression and individual drive suffer. The inspiration which comes to one man alone in the night or at dawn has given to the world of medicine the most fantastic discoveries. The flame of an idea glows dim when exposed before too many unseeing

> eyes. (I see the ghost of Banting.) Teams should be available (and money) to help the visionary haul his ideas through the maze of experiments, turning theory into fact. We need not fear; the boorish 'chief' is extinct in our society. It's men that make institutions — institutions don't make men!

There is an interesting footnote to Baltzan's Soviet trip.[3] Yom Kippur, the holiest of Jewish holidays, came round while he and Steinman were in Moscow, so they sought out a synagogue to take part in the traditional service. The synagogue was packed. After the service, Steinman told Baltzan that someone wished to speak to him. An elderly man approached wearing the white suit of an intern and addressed Baltzan in broken Yiddish.

"You are Dr. Balt-ZAWN from Kishinev," he said, using the broad "A" and putting the emphasis on the last syllable, the way Baltzan is pronounced in Europe.

Astounded at being recognized in such circumstances, Baltzan asked for an explanation. The man, it turned out, was one of scores of Soviet doctors who had been rounded up and jailed under the Stalin regime because they were suspected, for no good reason, of plotting to kill the Soviet leader. The man's cellmate while he was in prison was a poet from Kishinev named Baltzan, a second or third cousin of David Baltzan. The cousin had told the doctor the story of the Moishe Baltzan family's immigration to Canada, and the man recognized David years later under totally strange circumstances.

Baltzan, of course, had received considerable news coverage during his trip. As well, there was a strong family resemblance between David and the former cellmate of his new acquaintance.

The extraordinary meeting was doubly memorable for Baltzan: during it, he heard for the first time about two Kishinev relatives surviving the Nazi Holocaust — one a revolutionary poet, the other the secretary of the local Communist Party.

About a decade later Baltzan looked at more communist medicine, this time on a three-week tour of mainland China with Stuart Maddin, M.D., a colleague from Vancouver. Later they collaborated on a lengthy report, which was published[4] and given wide circulation. Among the many who studied the report was John Diefenbaker, who wrote to Baltzan specifically to comment on it:

> The article by yourself and Dr. Maddin . . . was read by Olive and me in detail. I never use the word 'fabulous' because it is so all-embracing that it can be applied to very few things. However, it does apply to that article, which reveals what Olive describes as 'the research of a working holiday.'

As with others who have studied medicine in China close up, Baltzan and Maddin were most fascinated by the combination of the ultra-modern with the traditional in technique, diagnosis and treatment:

> The re-emergence of a quaint practice in this golden age of medicine is sensational. Outstanding on the contemporary scene is the revival of traditional Chinese medicine. Chairman Mao Tsetung sensed the void of this art of healing for which Western medicine has not produced a substitute and restored it by edict. Generalissimo Chiang Kai-shek had created the vacuum by abolishing the ancient practice during his regime for the first time in its history of three millennia.

The doctors were intensely interested in almost everything they saw during what they described as

> . . . a zigzag tour from Canton to Peking, with daily or twice-daily visits to medical schools of both types, university and affiliated teaching hospitals, metropolitan general hospitals, including suburban, rural or commune clinics, health centres and research institutes.

They wrote, under the subtitle ''Morals and Medicine,'' of how syphilis was under such close control that only three primary infections had appeared in the preceding 12 months in the ''notorious'' port of Shanghai. Chinese authorities surprised them by explaining that the near eradication of the disease was due to the dissemination of information rather than introduction of antibiotics and chemotherapy.

Syphilis was not portrayed as the wages of sin or a source of shame, but rather a menace the state was obligated to eradicate:

> We, too, went a long way in this direction long ago by making the topic a parlour conversation piece. Then the therapeutic wonders appeared and pulled down the guards.

They did not see a department of psychiatry in any hospital they visited.

"Psychiatrists are not in demand. Parenthetically, on the other end figuratively speaking, the spectacle of haemorrhoid wards is not uncommon in some hospitals," they added with tongue in cheek.

The pace of life in China was unhurried, they found. Everyone seemed to be occupied, but no one was rushing. Physical fitness was a fetish with the population of all ages, its roots extending deep into the culture of the country.

> . . . the spirit of an intense nationalism is not a unique phenomenon in our times. The halo it bears is different. Its influence or the result of it on health problems is reminiscent of customs in ancient Grecian and Roman civilizations. The sacrifices are Spartan and, to paraphrase a Japanese saying, 'It may be a pleasure to give and not a joy to receive' in terms of the amenities of life. The guiding principle in all deeds is 'to help one's self in order to better serve the state.' This is in the reverse order of the Western precepts of socialism.

In the end, it appeared they were confused by the system of health care in China and they found more to criticize than to recommend. Their concluding thoughts took them back to the same issue with which they began their article, traditional medicine:

> The future course and shape of medicine (in China) will more likely be linked to their ancient culture with rapid adaptations of the modern scientific skills, rather than to the ideologies which divide us.

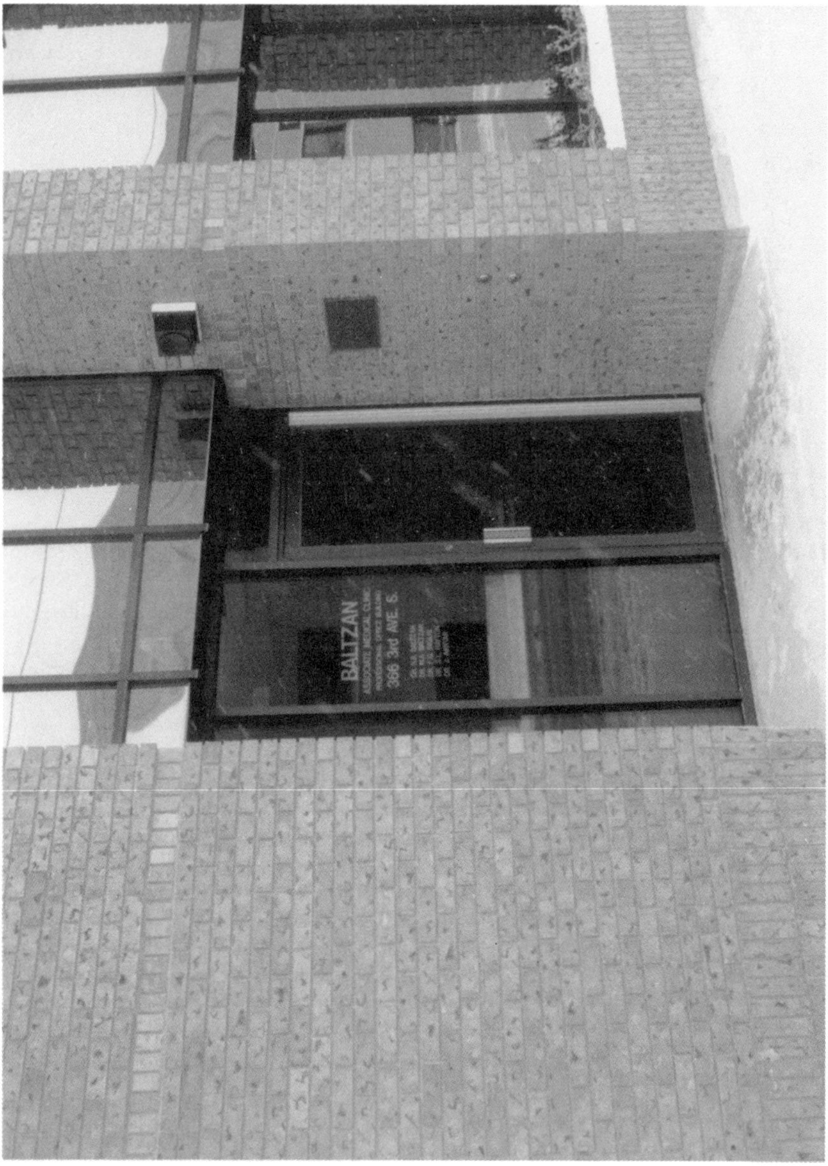

Entrance to the Baltzan Associate Medical Clinic. Photo courtesy Miriam Clemence

Chapter 8

The Consummate Professional

RICHARD BALTZAN followed in his father's footsteps, both as a specialist in internal medicine and as chief of the medical staff at St. Paul's Hospital in Saskatoon. When he was dismissed from the post in 1993 because of a disagreement with provincial and local health care politicians over who should decide the future of St. Paul's, a colleague paid him the ultimate compliment by telling him, "Your father would have been proud of you for standing on a principle."

Richard remembers his father with affection and respect. David Baltzan's towering intellect and devotion to principle set high standards for his three sons. Both the oldest son Marc and Richard (Donald died in 1956) speak of their father's high ethical standards often when they reflect on his life. So, for that matter, do most who knew him, professionally or otherwise.

His sons knew him best. They recall him as a parent with high expectations for his sons, and as a colleague with high professional standards. That is not to say he was a saint, and his sons respect his memory enough to be honest in their assessments. The man they remember was human. Marc reflects, for example, that his father "could be very arrogant at times."

"He was not your dedicated, 'I'll sacrifice everything for the sake of science' type of man,'' Richard recalls. ''He did work hard, but he liked his creature comforts. He liked to travel first class. He loved his Rolls.''

He was not a man to suffer fools gladly.

''He would speak his mind. He inspired loyalty among people, but he was not universally loved. Anybody that is in a senior position and has to make tough decisions makes some enemies along the way.''

If not universally loved, the David Baltzan whose memory is revered by his sons and many others, and who is thoroughly respected even by those with whom he disagreed, was universally regarded as a man of the highest integrity. As Richard puts it, his father was not a ''schemer politician,'' though he was skilled at dealing with people. ''He would be out front. He didn't play games.''

His long-time friend Emmett Hall, who chaired the board of St. Paul's Hospital for much of the time David Baltzan was both chief of staff and chief of the department of medicine, and who headed the royal commission on health care upon which Baltzan served, is blunt: ''When Dave Baltzan said it, it was so.''

Baltzan was heavily involved in the business world. He invested in shares and stocks and he and his brother invested in hotels and other property in Alberta, including a furniture store. He believed firmly that medicine and business should be kept separate, however, and was determined that the Baltzan name not be denigrated in any way, such as when a cousin sought to use the name in the operation of a furniture store.

David counselled his sons to conduct business activities in a city and province other than Saskatoon and Saskatchewan, where the Baltzan Clinic was located. He was displeased when they ignored his advice and for a time became owners of the Bessborough Hotel, the most prestigious in Saskatoon.

He applied the same ethical standards to medical business. At times, his ways were seen as too stiff-necked or rigid by other medical practitioners wishing to bend the rules.

''Father was one of the first to put the College of Physicians and Surgeons on the right track. You know, fee-splitting and under-the-table type payments and things. He wouldn't have any part of that. Everyone always knew where he stood on issues.''

Ernie Baergen knew David Baltzan both as a teacher and through the Saskatchewan Medical Association. Baergen retired in 1992 after serving 25 years as executive director of the S.M.A. He was a medical student taught by Baltzan when he was a clinical instructor at University Hospital in Saskatoon, one of many practising physicians who would take students around the wards. They would be taken in groups to the bedside where they were instructed in the technique of physical examination and the art of diagnosis, followed by discussions on treatment.

"He was known as a rather dramatic teacher," Baergen recalls. "He liked to do things with a flair." The students were fond of Baltzan because he seemed interested in them and dealt with them in a compassionate way. "He wasn't a tough teacher, as you might expect from his reputation."

Baltzan was not only known in teaching circles, but also in the realm of professional associations. The College of Physicians and Surgeons and the Saskatchewan Medical Association were both established early in the century, around the time the Province of Saskatchewan entered Confederation (1905). The two organizations functioned on parallel courses until 1937, when a conflict arose between them because of their overlapping functions[1] during a time when the Depression was making it difficult for each of them separately to send delegates to conferences.

It was David Baltzan, as president of the Saskatchewan Medical Association, who presided over a meeting in which it was decided that the S.M.A. would merge with the College of Physicians and Surgeons. The College thus became the sole representative body for doctors in the province, a situation that lasted, successfully for the most part, for 30 years.

In 1967, in a twist of fate, David's son Marc proposed that there should be two organizations again. For the first two years of the S.M.A's renewed existence, Marc followed his father's example and served as president. Around that time David Baltzan's own career began gradually to wind down. By the time Ernie Baergen took over the post, he had few dealings at all with David directly.

* * *

In the intervening years of only one association, the registrar of the College of Physicians and Surgeons had accumulated a substantial file on the outspoken internist. Much of the material had to do with Baltzan's work on two College committees. The College was also a clearing house for problems arising between individual practitioners, and between the College and doctors who transgressed the rules that guided professional conduct.

True to character, Baltzan was not in the least reluctant to speak out when the occasion demanded, as in the example of an exchange he had in 1937 with the head of the Saskatoon Tuberculosis Sanatorium, Dr. Harvey Boughton[2], when Boughton refused to provide Baltzan with clinical information on a patient who had been referred by another physician. Baltzan wrote to Boughton:

> You seemed quite annoyed on several occasions when we telephoned for information regarding patients you examined. It seems the referring doctor only is entitled to this information. I could hardly believe that this is true! I do not know where else such a rule is practised. It is ridiculous, obsolete and narrow provincialism. We ourselves are in exactly the same position regularly, almost daily, and I don't care at all what a referring doctor thinks, though I may be even more dependent on such good will than you as an institution are dependent — yet once I have an opinion it is open to anyone with the exception of such a person who is requiring it for meddlesome reasons, and that is where I draw the line.

Baltzan went on to cite specific cases where his clinic had freely given information, then added:

> In honest medicine there is no offense to the referring physician, there is co-operation with the second and it means harmony in so far as the involved patient [is concerned].
>
> . . . Your policy may keep you out of hot water with a narrow-minded referring physician (once in a long while) but every patient that we have to bluntly tell that you are withholding your findings and that we have to re-X-ray, re-test and cover the same ground again — thinks little of this system. He is rightfully prejudiced . . . I am writing this letter in the hope organized medicine may profit. I think your policy is bad.
>
> Surely this nonsense can stop without hardship on anybody and goodwill to all . . . if your policy remains fixed, let me know and we will never bother you again — I still can't believe it!

Boughton sent a copy of Baltzan's letter to the College, saying the Sanatorium staff had always taken the attitude that medical reports belonged only to referring physicians unless specifically instructed otherwise:

> In this instance, the patient was referred by a physician from outside Saskatoon, and the patient, after being at the Sanatorium, decided to consult Dr. Baltzan. Before we had an opportunity of reporting to the referring physician, Dr. Baltzan phoned the Sanatorium asking the results of our examination, and was met with my refusal to comply.
>
> We have always felt that any other attitude would be unethical, and we have maintained this stand . . . I would be glad to have the advice of the Council [of the College of Physicians and Surgeons].

Dr. J.G.K. Lindsay, registrar of the College, took the matter to a meeting of the Council a few weeks later. In a subsequent letter to Boughton, with a copy to Baltzan, the Council ruled:

> . . . the referring doctor should receive the report on a patient as has been the practice of the Sanatorium and Cancer Clinics in the past.

To that, the ever-eloquent Baltzan responded in scathing tones:

> Would you please record that the resolution referred to . . . is entirely beside the point. Of course the referring physician should receive a report. Whoever denied that well recognized principle!

Baltzan's point, of course, was that the resolution did not deal with the desirability of the information being made available to doctors other than the referring physician, so that patients would not have to be investigated all over again before obtaining another opinion.

> Surely to Heaven, if one is not ashamed of one's findings, and the Sanataria have a well-merited respect, can these findings not be available to any recognized doctor who has the patient's case under consideration at the moment?

> As the resolution reads, I object to having my name attached to an ambiguous statement and an irrelevant question.

A chastened registrar replied, saying he had "clumsily recorded the title to the resolution," and agreed to re-introduce the issue at the next Council meeting. The file does not contain the final disposition, if such there was.

Bureaucracies were favourite targets for Baltzan. A few months after his run-in with Boughton, he was writing to the registrar of the College again, this time about a provincial government policy under which municipal governments reimbursed doctors 25 percent of their fees for patients on relief and unable to pay. It was called the "necessitous care to relief recipients." But the public did not understand how the scheme worked.

> People are flocking in with municipal and government certificates for all sorts of work. A lot is pure luxury. Irrespectively their understanding is that the doctors are getting full compensation. Very few know that 25 percent is recognized. Even if this is not really true — (the limit is $100 if and when you get it.)

Baltzan called on Registrar Lindsay to make a press statement to clear up the misunderstanding, taking pains not to blame the individuals involved, since "they come innocently believing they are preferred customers and expect a lot."

The registrar referred Baltzan's letter to a health department authority in the hope a government statement would be made. Lindsay wrote:

> I believe pressure can be brought to bear this way, which would be reasonable in view of the tardiness with which the money is being paid for this emergency service.

These records and others like them taken from the files of the College demonstrate the straightforward responses Baltzan was known for. He continued to speak out.

A move by the College to adopt the Royal College's code of ethics on communications to the public, in which individual physicians were forbidden to speak out on medical subjects in favour of a view "from some organized and recognized medical society or association," brought him to the barricades with guns blazing.

A fierce defender of an individual's right to speak, Baltzan warned his colleagues, to no avail, of the dangers inherent in the proposed code. It included a provision that violators could be investigated as to their fitness to be licensed.

When a bureaucrat in the province's Medical Care Insurance Commission told a patient in error that David Baltzan was not entitled to a specialist fee because he was listed as a general practitioner, his wrath was quick and sure:

> I charge you with an act of gross and damaging misrepresentation . . . your action is libellous.

Needless to say, the sheepish recipient of the letter set matters straight post haste.

These examples illustrate Baltzan's forthright character. The bulk of the David Baltzan record with the College of Physicians and Surgeons chronicles his extensive work in the areas of education, professional conduct and medicine. He shared his wisdom and judgment generously. As well, the many honours he received over the years, both in connection with his medical practice and in his humanitarian work in the broader community, reflected well on the whole medical profession.

* * *

Speculating about what made his father who he was, Richard Baltzan draws on a period of about two years during his high school days. With his older brothers at McGill, their mother went to Montreal for extended periods to look after their needs while Richard and his father fended for themselves. They became very close during that period. Richard believes his father was drawn to medicine, the first in his family to take it up, for more than one reason.

Partly, he thinks, it was because medical practice was the epitome of service and accomplishment for a Jewish man of his era, and he was determined to be the best in whatever he did. Medicine also intrigued him intellectually. David had all the dexterity needed to be a surgeon, but surgery did not interest him. Rather it was "the game" of diagnosing disease and prescribing a treatment to help the afflicted that so fascinated him, as opposed to "the process" of cut and cure.

As a teenager, Richard learned through his close association with his father, and later as a colleague in medical practice, that David Baltzan took a great deal of pride in his work, his world travel, his recognition professionally. He was supremely self-confident and not a humble man.

Early in his career he combined ambition for success with a determination to stick to the highest standards of professional skill and ethics. Doubtless that accounted for his deep involvement over the years with professional associations, and for his efforts in the late 1920s, just as he was getting his own practice started, to found The Royal College of Physicians and Surgeons of Canada.

* * *

The national voluntary organization was established by a special act of Parliament in 1929, with David Baltzan as one of the charter members. Headquartered in Ottawa, its stated objectives are as follows:[3]

a) to further the excellence of professional training and the standards of practice in the various medical and surgical specialties in Canada;
b) to contribute to the improvement of health care of Canadians through the provision of designations for specialty trained physicians and surgeons, whereby it may be known that they are properly qualified;
c) to maintain a high standard of professional ethics, conduct and practice among medical and surgical specialists;
d) to encourage, assist and promote continuing medical education;
e) to initiate, encourage, support and extend interest in research in medicine and medical education;
f) to encourage, assist and promote the study of quantitative and qualitative aspects of specialized health care in Canada;
g) to encourage, assist and have continuing concern with health matters.

— Chapter 9 —

Working in the Community

SASKATOON was a small city of fewer than 45 000 when David Baltzan was establishing his medical practice and raising three young sons with his wife Rose.

The city had a Jewish community numbering about 500, most of whom lived on the west side. David's parents had also lived on the west side of the city, but when they married, David and Rose bought their first home on the east side in a newer area. As Marc and Richard Baltzan recall life in those days, the main reason for the concentration of Jewish families in one area of the city was economic. The land and housing in that section of the city were less costly than in the newer, developing areas. The west side was also where most of the small shops were located, many of which were run by members of the Jewish community, so there was also an element of convenience.

David and Rose were part of a Jewish community that actively supported a synagogue and a rabbi (when available). The recruiting of a rabbi and the non-stop business of fund-raising dominates the archival history of the city's Jewish community from that period.[1]

The extensive records list pledges and collections of $1, $5, sometimes $10. Each family gave what it could afford. David Baltzan's name appears regularly on the list of contributors, with the amount of his donations reflecting the times; shrinking during the struggle of the Depression years, growing again as the post-war years brought prosperity.

The early years, when anti-Semitism was on the rise and white supremacists, most notably the Ku Klux Klan, operated briefly in Saskatchewan, were obviously anxious times for Jewish groups in every community. In the late 1930s, the Saskatoon community raised money to help defend Jews everywhere against ultra-rightists and would-be fascists, who without hindrance preached hatred against a variety of identifiable minorities at one time or another: Jews, Roman Catholics, non-whites.

Local Jewish leaders received reports on hostile activities across the country by groups such as The National Unity Party, The Canadian Union of Fascists and The National Christian Party. In their turn, they reported on any local activity that threatened the community.

In 1939, one report suggested some 380 people in Saskatchewan had joined the National Unity Party, a quarrelsome amalgamation of several rightist splinter groups whose members decided to become followers of the infamous "Bobolink", the Quebec Fascist hate-monger Adrian Arcand.

Arcand claimed to be head of the National Unity Party at the time and used his publishing business in Quebec to spread propaganda and promote the myth that his organization was a country-wide movement. When the strutting Arcand was jailed along with some of his closest followers, the local anti-Semitism threat appeared to dissipate.

This pattern was much as had occurred on previous occasions, with the hate groups never coming close to being mainstream, as they claimed, or acquiring more than a handful of serious members. The Second World War, of course, was a call to arms for Jewish communities as word spread of the genocidal horrors in Europe.

The Baltzans themselves experienced no personal discrimination in the community, then or later, and they do not believe it was ever an issue in Saskatoon. Marc recalls only one episode, when his brother Donald got into a fight as a young boy over name-calling in the school yard.

Indeed, individuals such as David Baltzan were front and centre in many medical and non-medical community endeavours. Sid Buckwold, a member of a prominent business family, went on to become mayor, and later a Senator. Jack Goldenberg was the acknowledged leader of the Jewish community and a prominent figure in the city as a whole. There was little to evoke the stereotypes or old hatreds that led to anti-Semitism elsewhere.

Richard speculates that his father may have encountered anti-Semitism while he was living and studying in Vienna for two years. The time of his tenure, the late 1920s and the early 1930s, coincides with the rise of Nazi leader Adolf Hitler in Germany and Austria, though neither Richard nor Marc recall actually hearing their father talk about any such experience.

David and Rose went to the synagogue regularly in the early years and their two oldest sons, Marc and Donald, had their bar mitzvahs. David did not always see eye-to-eye with the leaders in the Jewish community, however, and he had disagreements with other members of the synagogue.

When a new synagogue was built, an egalitarian seating arrangement was implemented, which meant that the seat that David had inherited on his father's death was no longer his by right. From that point on, his attendance at services became irregular.

When it came time for Richard's bar mitzvah, the rabbi told Baltzan his son had been skipping Hebrew classes to play ball and therefore was not ready for the ceremony. David was angry, but Marc and Donald intervened and convinced their father that Richard was not interested. David relented. Thereafter he lost interest altogether in the synagogue.

Both surviving sons recall that their mother continued to observe religious custom for a time — lighting candles on Friday nights, for example — but that, too, dropped off.

* * *

David Baltzan's vision of a just society went beyond the confines of one group, dedicated though he was to the Jewish community. The fledgling Canadian Council of Christians and Jews and the old established B'nai B'rith spoke more to his broad concept of multiculturalism, honed, perhaps, by his world travels and his first-hand experiences with people of many colours and ethnic origins.

It was that sort of philosophy that led him to work directly with the Council of Christians and Jews. In the mid-1950s, he had become widely known for this activity and was honoured at a ceremony in Calgary, where he received the council's Human Relations Award. In the words

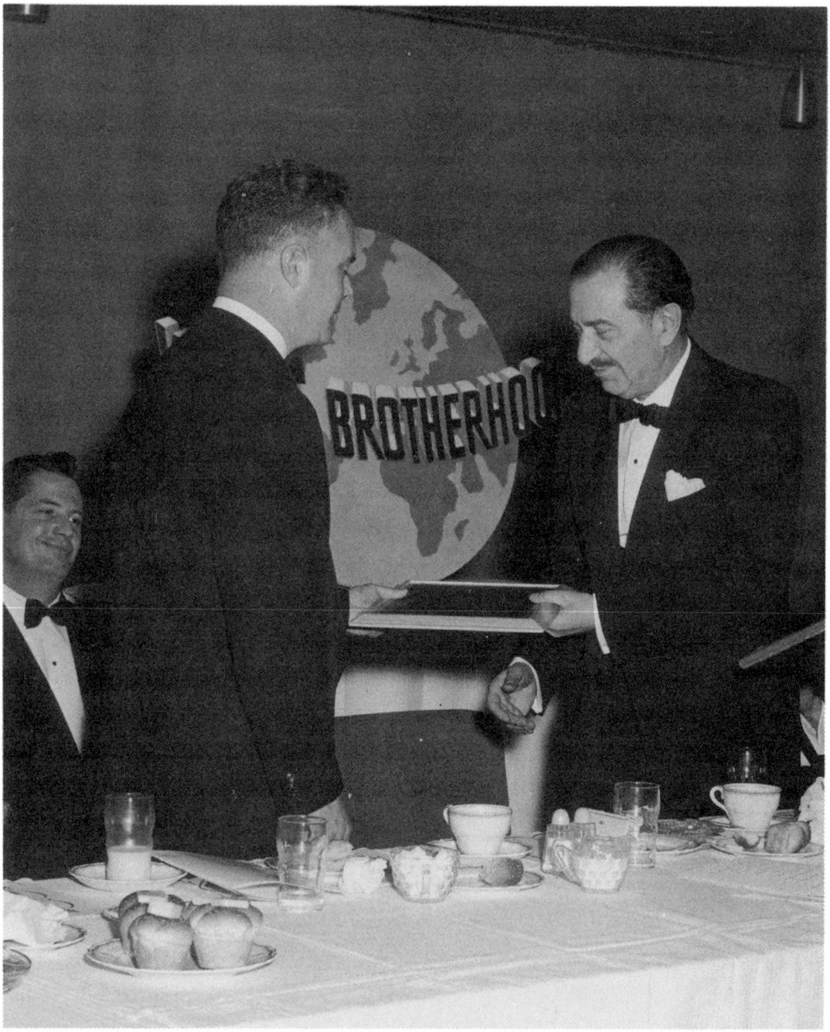

David Baltzan receiving an award in Calgary from the Canadian Council of Christians and Jews, presented by newspaper publisher Max Bell (left)

of Calgary Herald publisher Max Bell, who presented the award, David had attempted to write "the enduring prescription of brotherhood into the hearts of all mankind."

In his acceptance speech, Baltzan exhorted others in the Council:

> . . . to extend their efforts to the promotion of world fellowship rather than the narrower conception of brotherhood between Christians and Jews. If it is good for Christians and Jews, it should be good for other religions, races and cultures.

In 1979, his work was honoured further with the establishment at St. Thomas More College in the University of Saskatchewan of the Dr. David M. Baltzan Lectureship in Judaic Studies.

Baltzan's aspirations for world Jewry never wavered. He made that clear in a newspaper article he wrote after he attended the Seventh World Assembly of the Israeli Medical Association as a delegate of the American Physicians Fellowship. The gathering, planned three years in advance, was held little more than a month after the end of the Six Day War that rocked the Middle East and the world.

In the article, Baltzan called it the Blitz and Bliss war because it had been so fast and furious and, when he visited Israel, the populace was so calm, almost in a state of bliss at having dispatched their ancient enemies.

In the wake of the conflict, after viewing some of the damage, he wrote hopefully:

> With peace and a humane approach, stabilization can occur. There must never be a Gaza strip fiasco again where about 200 000 people were segregated, subsisting on the dole from the UN for nearly 20 years. They were hostages for political barter where the young were being trained in Egypt for a war of revenge.

* * *

Baltzan had an eye and an ear for those in need and for injustice. He demonstrated over and over again an unusual ability to bridge differences between people and ideas. At a time when conventional wisdom supported a punitive approach to crime with little time for rehabilitation, Baltzan made a name for himself by publicly supporting the John Howard

Society. Yet he maintained a rapport with the business community and conservatives (both small and large C), and became one of the most effective fund-raisers when St. Paul's Hospital had to come up with a substantial portion of the cost of its rebuilding program.

He worked, too, for United Way in Saskatoon.

His early work as the first director of the Saskatoon Cancer Clinic was, in large measure, also a voluntary position.

His years of serving as a consultant to the tuberculosis sanatorium could hardly have returned anything close to what his services earned him as one of the province's foremost medical specialists.

His work with the board administering the Queen Elizabeth Canadian Fund for Research on Diseases of Children was, of course, voluntary.

The greatest unpaid public service undertaking of his career, however, was his work on the royal commission studying health care in Canada. Emmett Hall, who headed the commission, doubted if Baltzan's expenses were even adequately covered, to say nothing of what it cost him by way of lost income while he was absent from his clinic at commission hearings, or travelling outside Canada to investigate health systems in other countries.

* * *

David Baltzan served in the two top medical posts in St. Paul's Hospital for many years. No one really seemed to find it surprising that a Jewish doctor should become a legend for his work in a Roman Catholic hospital, or that his sons should follow in his footsteps, all without any friction attributable to religious differences.

Indeed, as Richard Baltzan pointed out, the chief of staff in a major hospital inevitably makes enemies. But whatever conflicts David Baltzan engaged in, they were resolved without resort to anti-Semitism. He was one of the leaders in the hospital while it went through a long period of uncertainty as to its future, up to the final decision to replace the old building.

The history of St. Paul's written by the Saskatoon author Sally Clubb[2] relates how the hospital's managers began the decade of the 1950s making plans to enlarge the 50-year-old facility with the addition of upwards of 100 beds in a new wing, bringing its capacity up to about 370.

Baltzan was appointed to a three-member committee — along with board chairman Emmett Hall and board member Judge McKercher — to start the ball rolling. It didn't roll very far, unfortunately, in spite of signs that the city's three hospitals would soon be unable to handle their increasing loads.

Teaching requirements, a growing population in the city and the far-flung northwest part of the province served by Saskatoon's hospitals, together with rapid advances in medical science, combined to create an urgent need for beds and more modern facilities.

The architects argued that the building was old and at the end of its useful life. If there was to be an addition, the original structure would have to be renovated at a cost of some $300 000, and even then the building would barely be adequate.

When the architects then pointed out that the best solution would be to build a whole new hospital, the provincial and federal governments were brought in. By that time, Tommy Douglas's CCF was in power in Saskatchewan and John Diefenbaker's Conservatives held sway at the national level. Joint policy on hospital construction was practically non-existent. There was no clear delineation of responsibility and buck-passing was the order of the day. Governments are slow to act at the best of times: this time in particular was not a good one for getting things done.

The records do not reveal exactly who did what in the end, though obviously the role of the three-member committee was crucial. The work went on over a period of almost 10 years before tenders were let and construction of a modern institution began.

Provincial and federal governments both changed their stripes, and in the course of doing so, new health care policies were invented. No doubt all the negotiating and political skills David Baltzan had developed were called into use. Correspondence with John Diefenbaker during this time reveals guarded exchanges between the two.

In April 1959, for example, Baltzan wrote to Diefenbaker to say he had heard that the provincial government was stalling on attaching its signature to a particular phase of the hospital deal that was currently on the table. In an underlined passage he wrote:

> The excuse is a delayed reply to some letters sent to Ottawa. I think it is a bluff. Could you pass this enquiry on and have someone write to me privately.

A week or so later, Diefenbaker's private secretary wrote back in a letter prominently marked "Personal and Confidential":

> We have had the question of St. Paul's Hospital looked into and I wish to advise you that apparently there has been no official move on the part of the Province to take the matter up with Federal authorities.

Whether that really answered Baltzan's question can only be a matter for conjecture. It is probable that it was just one of many such letters he wrote to friends in both camps — Baltzan and Premier Douglas were on good terms as well — in an effort to keep the process moving.

The architects' recommendations eventually won the day. By the mid-1950s, all sides agreed that building onto St. Paul's was not practical. It only remained to work out who would pay to replace the ageing institution completely. After a few more years of skirmishing it was agreed that the province would pay just over $3 million, the federal government just under $1 million and the Grey Nuns about $1 million. For that sum, a new 332-bed hospital would be constructed.

It was a red-letter day when the *Saskatoon StarPhoenix* reported, 18 April 1961, that the Sisters of Charity (Grey Nuns) had announced that tenders had been called and construction was expected to start in mid-summer. It was hoped the new hospital would be occupied before the end of 1962.

David Baltzan was just one of the many hospital representatives at the new building's opening ceremonies. He said in a note to John Diefenbaker some time later that he was content to remain in the background and let the politicians occupy the limelight: all he wanted was the new hospital. The comment typified Baltzan's approach to his community work. For an individual who moved easily in lofty circles, who was the recipient of many honours of a national and international nature, who spoke off-handedly of meeting the Pope and who socialized in the upper echelons of government, he seemed curiously uncomfortable at the idea of giving any appearance of putting himself forward.

David Baltzan's sense of service to his community and the wider world was such that he eschewed recognition. Nevertheless, it is a curious fact that no local streets, parks, swimming pools or other civic amenities bear his name as a memorial, yet recognition has been freely bestowed upon many others who, although doubtless worthy, contributed a good deal less.

— Chapter 10 —

The Family Man

DAVID BALTZAN's work was his consuming passion for most of his life. The effect that this had on the Baltzan family life was predictable. Richard, the youngest of the three sons born to David and Rose, recalls that his father had little time for him and his brothers when they were children. Nor had he time for their mother, much to her chagrin.

Rose married David in 1927, just as he was setting up his own practice after turning down an offer to teach in the College of Medicine in Edmonton, where Rose's family lived. For Rose, there was no thought of a job or career outside the home. Although that was not uncommon for many women of her time, those who married doctors tended to be "homebodies" even more than most. They lived their lives through their husbands' dedication to others — often despite the fact that, for the members of the male-dominated medical profession themselves, "others" seemed to include everyone but their own wives and children.

The year that the stock market crashed, 1929, saw the birth of their first child, Marcel, known for most of his life as Marc. Donald arrived in 1932 and Richard in 1935. For the most part, Rose raised the boys on her own. She also reached out to her sister, who was married to David's brother and who fell prey to Parkinson's Disease in 1937.

When her sister ceased to be able to care for her family, Rose looked

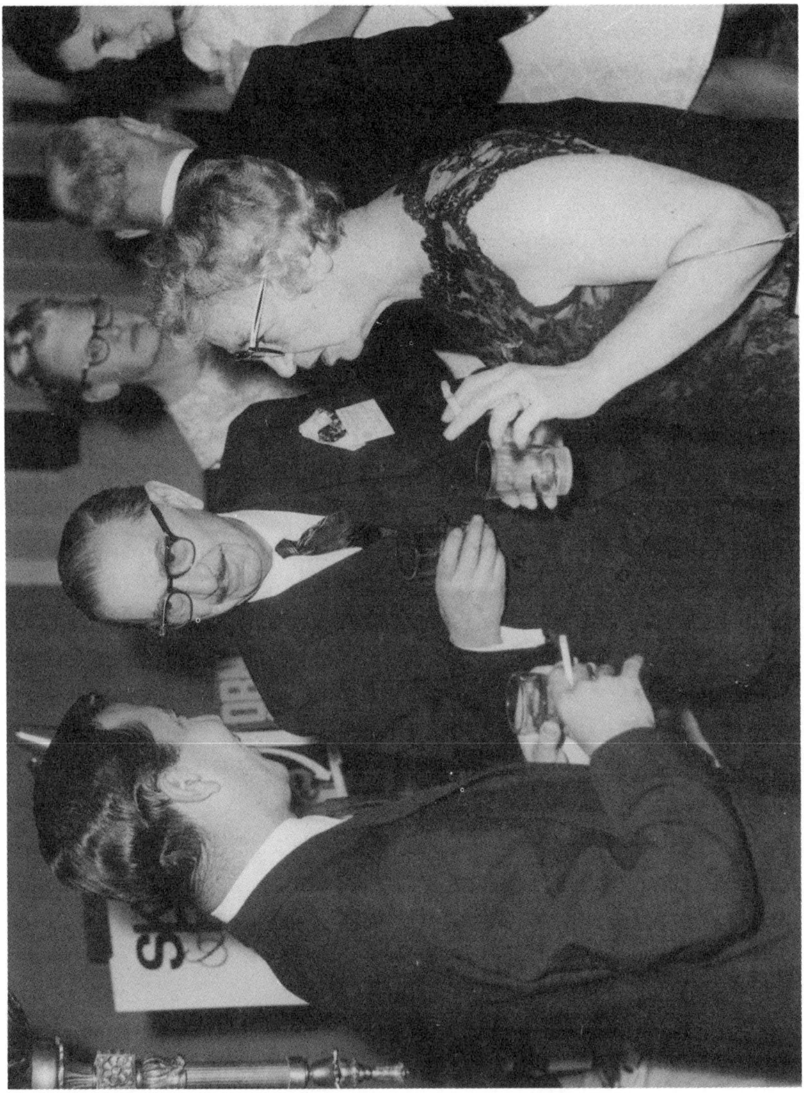

A social occasion in Saskatoon: Richard Baltzan (left), David and Rose

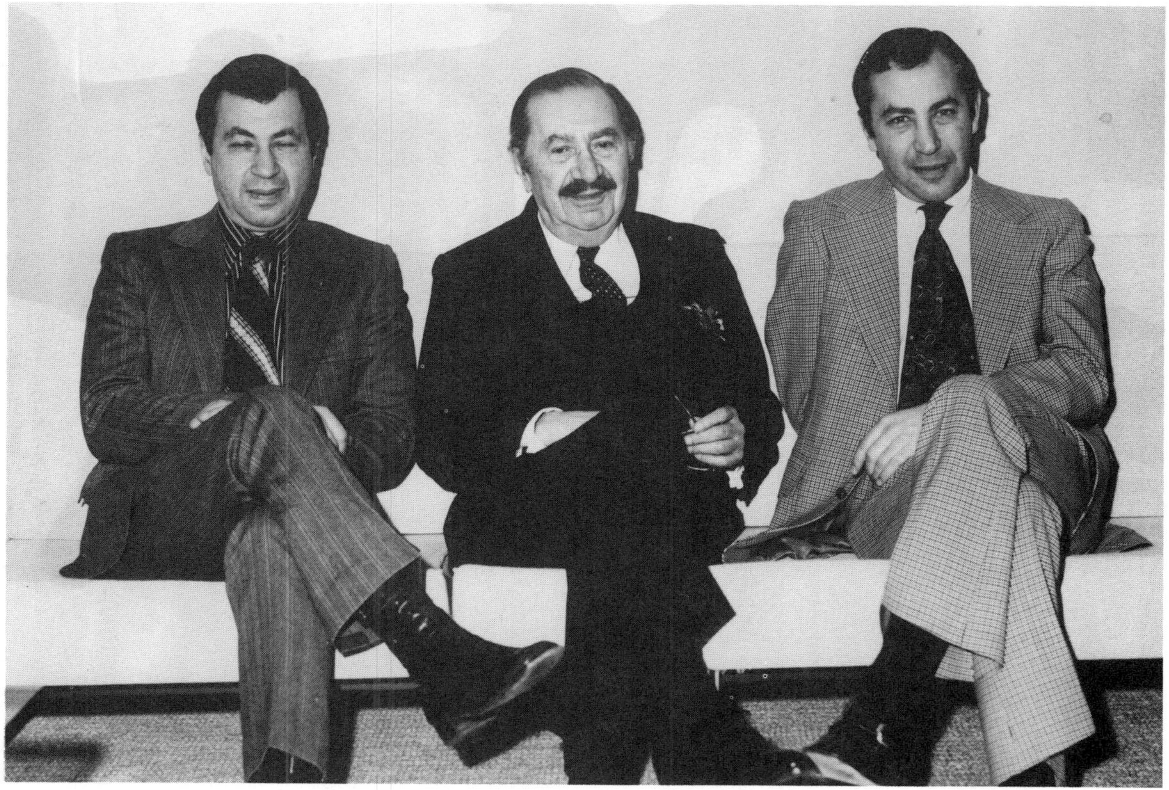

Marc (left), David and Richard

after the stricken woman's two children much of the time and treated them as *de facto* siblings (they were, after all, double cousins, or genetic brothers and sisters) for her own three sons.

In later life, one friend recalls, Rose was fond of showing off her own "MD" — "Mother of Doctors" — certificate, bestowed upon her by her family.

Despite her dedication, Rose did manage several outside interests as well. She developed a talent for oil painting. She was a founding member of the National Council of Women. She was among the first 10 members of the Saskatoon Co-operative Association and was active on the Council of Women in Saskatoon as well as in Hadassah, the community organization for Jewish women. She was an excellent hostess at the elegant gatherings she and David held periodically in their home. She was a supporter of the arts in the community: she is remembered in particular for her appreciation of music.

For the most part, however, day-to-day life was a constant round of looking after the house and organizing the lives of her husband and children, especially in the early years. David worked late almost every night, rarely going to bed before 2:00 a.m. and seldom waking before 10:00 a.m.

Although Marc and Richard both remember their mother as the one they looked to for care and attention, it was David's influence that set the standards for their behaviour. Whether he was home or not, his presence was felt.

He did not believe in corporal punishment. His sons speak of his quiet way in his dealings with them and, most importantly, of not wanting to earn his wrath or disappointment. It was the custom of the time for families to be organized in a hierarchical system, with the father firmly in charge. Where in other families such an arrangement frequently resulted in parent/child conflicts ending with the infliction of punishment from on high, David Baltzan had a different way of dealing with disagreements between father and son.

"Father had this technique of inducing what we'd call guilt trips now; of exerting control in a very subtle manner."

"He never struck any of the children. Never once. Hardly ever raised his voice to any of the children."

Nevertheless, David had his ways.

Marc remembers a quiet, understated authority figure, one unquestionably in charge. He chuckles at recollections of the few times he got into his father's bad books. In his teenage years, for example, when he had his own charge accounts for necessities, he decided he just had to have a Second World War surplus flight jacket, which were all the rage at the time. Without asking his father, he bought one for about $13. He knew before he even got home that he was going to be in big trouble.

''Did I catch hell because it wasn't authorized!''

Marc seldom abused his charge account privileges after that, because he knew that any time he went too far, he would be called to account to explain his profligacy.

Donald, or Donny, the middle son who died of cancer in 1988, was an ''offbeat devil'' in Marc's recollection. He was the only one of the three who was inclined to violate curfews and otherwise bend his father's rules.

One night when Donny was in high school and had stayed out past his curfew, David decided to sit up and wait for him so that he could have a talk with his wayward son. Eventually he grew weary and went to bed, leaving a note that said, ''Donald, please wake me up when you get home.'' The unsuspecting youth, thinking some family crisis had arisen, shook David awake.

''Father, Father, what's going on?''

''Oh, so you're home now. Thank you for waking me up.''

David then read his son the riot act.

''I don't know if Donald ever came in late again,'' Marc said, ''but if he did, he didn't read any notes after getting suckered like that. Father got a good sleep and still got Donny. Pretty good strategy for an old guy.''

Neither Marc nor Richard remember ever having the notion spelled out for them, but they both clearly recall that they all knew from an early age that they were expected to become doctors. At different points, however, Richard and Donald both very briefly contemplated careers outside of medicine.

For the latter it happened when the three brothers were at university in Montreal together and Donald had just been accepted into medicine, having finished his arts degree. He told the other two that on considering the matter, he had decided he no longer wanted to follow the medical path. The three brothers stayed up all night, talking. By morning, Donald had changed his mind.

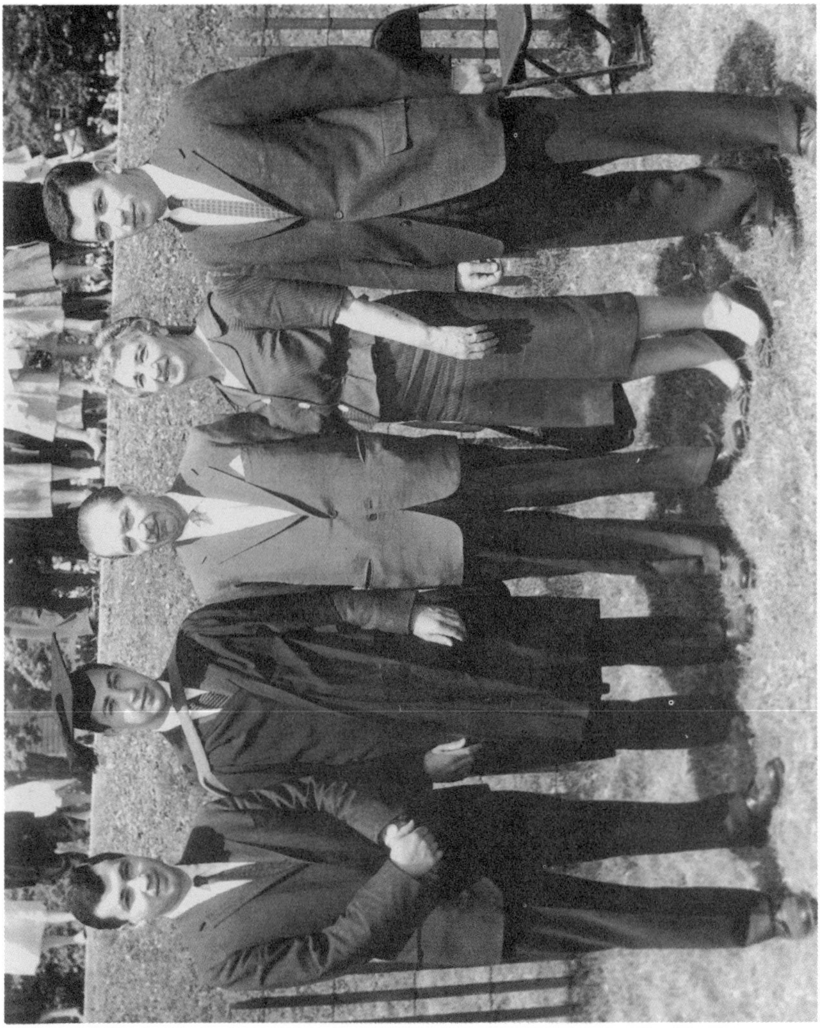

The Family: Marc (left), Richard (in graduation robes), David, Rose and Donald

He became a surgeon, was very happy and had a highly successful career.

Richard's "semi-crisis" (as he called it) occurred when he was in his third year of medicine. He was, in his own words, "a pretty good hockey player" — good enough to be invited to try out for the New York Rangers. It was a prestigious if not particularly lucrative offer in those days of the six-team National Hockey League. Richard, as a keen athlete, was drawn to the idea of being a pro hockey player. He knew a basketball player in third-year medicine who played for the New York Knicks. If pro basketball, why not hockey?

He finally broached the subject to his father.

"We had a long chat. He sat me down, and he said, 'It's your decision, but your chances of making it in the NHL, and making it big, are negligible.' Actually, they probably were not that bad. He wasn't belittling me. It was just a very serious conversation, and at the end of it I chose medicine. I have never regretted my decision."

Siblings often offer different recollections of their parents. Obviously, such is not the case here. Richard's memories clearly echo those of Marc, only more so, since it is Richard above all who has the most enduring memories of David Baltzan as a father. He was the only one of the three sons to spend long periods alone with him during the teenage years. With Rose making extended trips to Montreal to care for Donald and Marc while they attended school there, David and Richard were thrown on each other's company.

"It was when I was in Grade 11 and Grade 12. I really had a companionship with him, a one-on-one father/son relationship."

Among the things Richard came to understand about the man for whom he has such deep respect were the motives that drove him in his work. He came to the conclusion that his father had entered medicine because of the huge intellectual challenge it posed. The technical side of medicine did not fascinate David nearly as much as the discovery of the causes of disease and the search for ways to treat patients effectively.

It was a precious time for Richard, all the more so when the memory of it helped sustain him through the bad times of David's affliction with Alzheimer's. Both Marc and Donald were away when David's increasing difficulties with memory severely restricted him in his work and other activities.

Richard recalls the painful times when his father would experience the terrible frustration of his illness and rail against his limitations. After a lifetime of being in charge, of enjoying the resources of a prodigious memory and an exceptional intellectual capacity, Alzheimer's was a bitter fate for David and for those who loved him.

When it became impossible for Rose to care for him at home, she and the rest of the family endured the anguish of admitting him to an institution, where Richard visited him faithfully twice a week, sitting by his side while David talked to him in Yiddish, believing Richard to be his brother.

* * *

Eight years after David's death, it was not his decline but the legacy of his life's work that his sons recalled.

The Baltzan Clinic is a large, well-appointed facility occupying the second floor of a building the Baltzans own in downtown Saskatoon. The practice is almost exclusively by referral, apart from a few older patients and close friends. Originally, David's practice was both primary care and referral. Internal medicine as a specialty was so rare when he started out that it took a while to establish the referral side of the practice.

It was David's ambition to have his sons as partners. He had realized his dream by the mid-1960s, with Marc and Richard as specialists in internal medicine, like their father, and Donald as the surgeon of the group.

Altogether, in David's time, over a dozen specialists worked in the practice, which helped countless patients over the years and gained a reputation across Saskatchewan and beyond.

The clinic was only part of David Baltzan's life's work.

Many who knew him well believe David's role with the Hall Commission in the 1960s, which was ultimately responsible for the system of medicare the country enjoys still, was one of his most important accomplishments, and was recognized as such by David himself. With his work on the commission, he believed he had served the public and the profession well.

Marc and Richard believe that their father's "firsts" were also vitally important to him as agents in the struggle to advance medicine.

Among these, first and foremost, was the fact that he was the first specialist in internal medicine to practise in the province. He was also the first doctor to introduce the electrocardiogram, and quite possibly the first to use an X-ray machine. He was among the first in the medical profession to link smoking to heart disease, based on his own extensive clinical research. He wrote a textbook for nurses in training. He took a prominent part in the discovery and identification of a haemoglobin factor that had been unknown up to that time, and in so doing helped many who appeared to suffer from cyanosis — the so-called "blue baby" condition — but who in fact did not have a congenital heart abnormality, once believed to be its sole cause.

David Baltzan worked tirelessly to refine the process of diagnosing disease, an effort for which he was recognized by his peers in the city and province, contributing substantially to his consulting practice. He was in the vanguard of diagnosticians, a relatively new concept in the early days of his medical practice. He is widely remembered for the lengths to which he would go to make and stand behind a diagnosis.

* * *

Fred Mendel, one of Saskatoon's greatest benefactors and best-known businessmen, wrote in his memoirs[1] how a consultation with Baltzan in 1940 was the start of a long and close friendship.

Mendel was a dynamo of a man whose five-foot, one-inch (155 cm) stature cast a long shadow on two continents. He had made a couple of fortunes in pre-war Europe buying and selling livestock, importing Czarist currency after the Russian revolution and reviving and operating the meat packing business he and his siblings inherited from their father in Germany.

He secured a patent for a ham-curing process and by 1938 had established 15 meat-packing plants around Eastern Europe. Then in 1939, recognizing the dangers posed by the Nazis, he and his family left the Mendel meat-packing empire behind and moved to New York. Finding little there to inspire them, they turned their eyes toward Canada and moved to Montreal.

While living in Montreal, Mendel began to experience chest pains. He was under extreme stress, worrying about the outbreak of war in Europe, the fate of his business empire, the loss of his European assets and the uncertainty of the future. He consulted a heart specialist, one of the best in Montreal and a fellow of the Royal College of Physicians and Surgeons of Canada. The specialist admitted him to the Royal Victoria Hospital for observation and eventually diagnosed his condition as serious heart disease. Mendel was advised to avoid heavy work and worry, bad news indeed.

"It was like a sentence of death."

Driving on the streets of Montreal, despondent over his condition, he heard the famous speech by Winston Churchill, in which the master statesman exhorted his people to ". . . fight on the beaches, fight on the landing fields . . . we shall never surrender."

Mendel was rejuvenated.

"My spirits soared," he wrote.

He immediately packed up, and with his wife Claire and their daughter Eva, headed west. In Saskatoon the Mendels took up residence in the Bessborough Hotel, the city's finest. Claire asked the hotel staff to call a doctor to see Fred. Baltzan was summoned.

> That was when I first met Dr. David Baltzan, a fine physician who became a close friend. Like most Saskatonians, who categorized us as refugees, Dr. Baltzan was surprised to find us living in an apartment in the Bessborough, one of the leading hotels in Western Canada. He was surprised as well that, after his professional call, Claire sent flowers to his home. Dr. Baltzan examined me and announced that I showed no signs whatever of heart disability and that I had nothing to worry about. When I asked whether I should continue my long hours of work, he said, "You can do anything you wish to." I salute him as the man who restored my confidence, with advice I have honoured ever since.

A twist on this story,[2] which illustrates Baltzan's tenacity and the lengths to which he would go in his diagnoses, has it that Mendel ended up wondering just precisely what to believe about his chest pains. When he found out, Baltzan, having heard of his patient's love of horses and horseback riding — he had owned a large racing stable in Europe and was intensely interested in the sport — promptly suggested that Mendel put his condition to the test by going to Banff, a place of high altitude with less available oxygen, and taking a horse out for a gallop. Mendel took his advice, experienced no symptoms and returned to Saskatoon convinced.

Mendel lived life to the full, dying in 1976 at the age of 88, having overcome financing and other obstacles to establish Intercontinental Packers, a business that became the fourth largest in Canadian meat packing circles. Among his many other activities, he endowed the Mendel Art Gallery, a national treasure house of the works of, among others, Canadians during the Depression years.

A family friend tells another story about Baltzan's work in heart disease. David had trouble getting on the register at Saskatoon's City Hospital in the very early days of his practice, blocked, so the story goes, by the president of the University of Saskatchewan, who happened to be a doctor and the city's best known heart specialist.

Then the president was smitten with heart disease himself and found himself reaching out to the young internist for help. Whether Baltzan's attentions were life-saving or not, the patient responded well to the treatment he received. Baltzan's name was placed on the register at City Hospital.

One piece of advice David Baltzan was fond of giving others in the profession was that their greatest consultant was the library. He accumulated a large private medical library during his years of practice which he used extensively in his research. He bequeathed the collection to the University of Saskatchewan as the Baltzan Medical Canadiana Library.

''More than anything else,'' says Marc of his father, ''he was his own man. He stood up and fought for what he believed to be right, whether it was popular or unpopular.''

* * *

David Baltzan did not ''go gentle into that good night.''[3]

As the poet Dylan Thomas urged, he did ''rage, rage against the dying of the light,'' the light of his intelligence, the towering intellect which was gradually eroded as Alzheimer's took its insidious course. Only close family members know the full extent of his frustration and its manifestation.

Those who had been his colleagues were aware that David knew his fate, however, and they watched him resist it with all the strength he could muster.

The disintegration that dragged so forceful a mind to its death on 15 June 1983 was an irony overridden by his achievements in and out of medicine: his supremacy in the diagnosis and treatment of heart disease; his reputation as a consulting internist which resulted in the compilation of more than 100 000 case histories over his years in practice; his work with the Hall Commission; his dedication to bridging the cultural and religious gaps between nations and peoples.

It is unlikely that he would have been impressed with all the praise levelled at him on his death, or that he would have wished to have his life defined by any statistical accounting. David Baltzan was ever the restless seeker. In his only gesture towards recording his memoirs, a brief outline which he completed at about the same time the Alzheimer's was making itself felt, he saw himself as a frontiersman, one who pushed at the limits, whether in medicine or the complexities of human intolerance.

His satisfactions in medical practice came in the chase, not the capture.

He was a straightforward, predictable, uncomplicated man. Perhaps he gave the best indication of how he wished to be regarded when, as an honoured guest at a Roman Catholic Mass after his retirement, he addressed the congregation. He spoke briefly, relying upon the clichés called upon on such occasions, then summed up his feelings simply.

"I just appreciate being accepted for what I am."

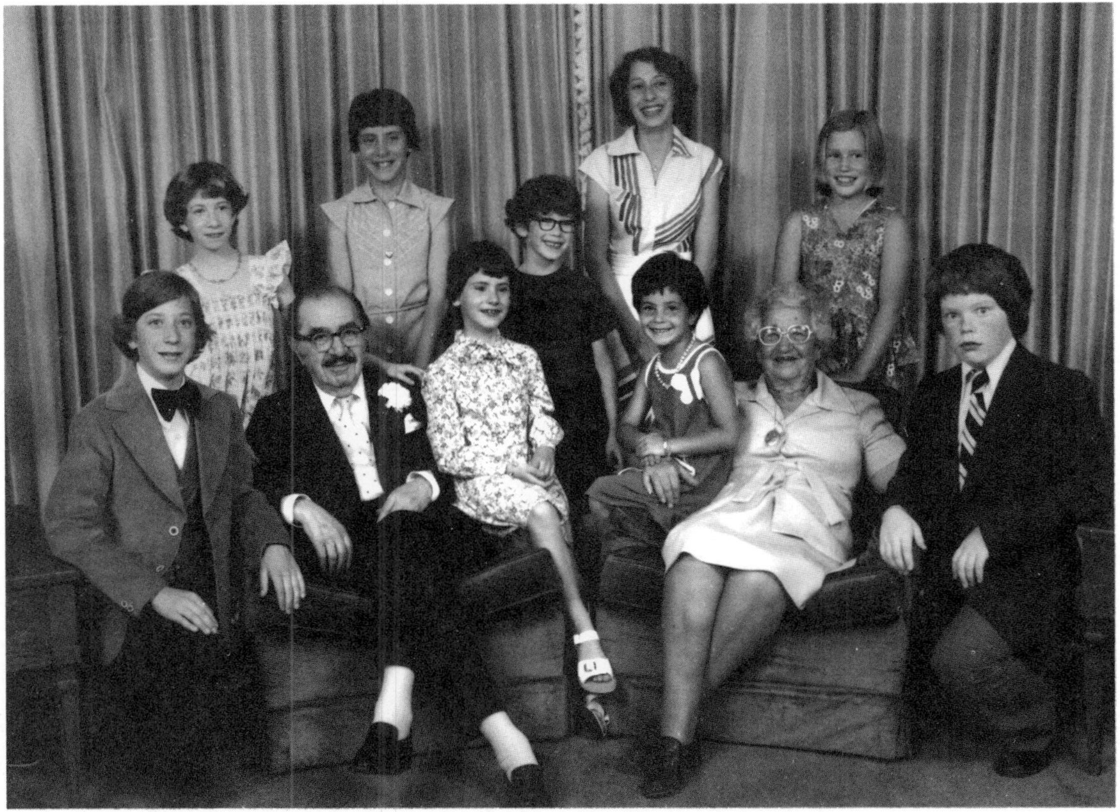

David and Rose Baltzan with their grandchildren

— Appendices —

Appendix I

David Mortimer Baltzan, M.D., F.R.C.P.(C), F.A.C.P.

Honours and Appointments

Professional and academic posts:

1. Chief of Staff, St. Paul's Hospital
2. Chief, Department of Medicine, St. Paul's Hospital
3. Professor of Clinical Medicine, University of Saskatchewan
4. Consultant in Medicine, University Hospital, University of Saskatchewan
5. Consultant in Medicine, Saskatoon City Hospital
6. Consultant in Medicine, Canadian National Railways
7. Consultant in Medicine, Tuberculosis Sanatorium, Saskatoon
8. First Clinical Director, Saskatchewan Cancer Clinic
9. President, Saskatchewan Medical Association
10. President, Academy of Medicine of Saskatchewan

Academic committee activities:

1. Chairman educational committee, Saskatchewan College of Physicians and Surgeons of Saskatchewan.
2. Member, Central Health Services Committee of Saskatchewan.

3. Member, University of Saskatchewan Post Graduate & Residency Committee.
4. Member, Committee on Continuation Studies, College of Medicine, University of Saskatchewan.
5. Chairman, Medical Advisory Board, St. Paul's Hospital.

Allied professional organizational bodies:

1. Vice-President, Saskatchewan Heart Foundation.
2. Member, Canadian Heart Foundation.
3. Member, Advisory Board, Society for the Chronically Ill.
4. Board Member, Queen Elizabeth II Canadian Fund to Aid in the Research of the Diseases of Children.

Medical societies:

1. Canadian Medical Association.
2. American Medical Association.
3. British Medical Association.
4. Councillor and Founder Canadian Heart Association.
5. Member, New York Academy of Science
6. Society of International Medicine of Canada.
7. Executive, Academy of Internal Medicine of Saskatchewan.

Non-professional associations:

1. Regional President, John Howard Society.
2. National Director, Council of Christians and Jews.
3. Western Vice-President, Canadian Jewish Congress.
4. President, Bnai B'rith.
5. Member, Advisory Board, United Appeal Saskatoon.

Recognitions:

1. Life Member of St. John's of Jerusalem.
2. Member, Canadian Authors Association.
3. Coronation Medal King George VI
4. Human Relations Award, Canadian Council of Christians and Jews.
5. Honorary Doctor of Laws, University of Saskatchewan.

Participation in foreign programs:

1. First World Heart Congress, paper read at Sorbonne.
2. Inter-American Heart Congress, paper read at Buenos Aires.
3. Canadian delegate, World Brotherhood, Brussels.
4. International Congress of Internal Medicine, Stockholm.

Endowments:

1. Baltzan Medical Canadiana Library, University of Saskatchewan.
2. Scholarship, Nutana Collegiate, Saskatoon.
3. Scholarship, Hebrew University, Jerusalem, Israel.
4. Lectureship in Judaic Studies, St. Thomas More College, University of Saskatchewan.

Appendix II

Publications by David Mortimer Baltzan

1. Baltzan, D.M., Digitalis administration. *Can. Med. Assoc. J.* May: 527-533, 1933.
2. Idem. A significant sign in coronary occlusion. Can. Med. Assoc. J. November: 538-539, 1933.
3. Idem. The management of the cardiac case. *Can. Med. Assoc. J.* September: 281-286, 1935.
4. Idem. A hepato-cerebral syndrome (Wilson's Disease). *Can. Med. Assoc. J.* May: 544-545, 1936.
5. Idem. Pituitary cachexia. *Can. Med. Assoc. J.* January: 64-66, 1937.
6. Idem. Experience with fifty-seven brucellosis infections in Saskatchewan. *Can. Med. Assoc. J.* March: 258-262, 1937.
7. Idem. Diagnosis of some major vascular accidents. *Can. Med. Assoc. J.* January: 45-49, 1938.
8. Idem. The treatment of angina pectoris. *Can. Med. Assoc. J.* April: 387-388, 1939.
9. Idem. Bronchomoniliasis in Saskatchewan. *Can. Med. Assoc. J.* September: 224-228, 1940.
10. Idem. *Principles of Internal Medicine: a course for nurses*. Toronto. Ryerson Press, pp. 398, (c) 1945.
11. Idem. Procedure in the treatment of heart disease. *Can. Med. Assoc. J.* 53: 150-156, 1945.

12. Idem. A simplified plan of prescribing for adult diabetes. *Can. Med. Assoc. J.* 57: 54-58, 1947.
13. Idem. and Sugarman, H. Hereditary cyanosis. *Can. Med. Assoc. J.* 62: 348-350, 1950.
14. Idem. The present status of the medical treatment of hyperthyroidism. *Can. Med. Assoc. J.* 62: 439-443, 1950.
15. Sugarman, H. and Baltzan, D.M. Primary splenic neutropenia with rheumatoid arthritis (Felty's syndrome). *Can. Med. Assoc. J.* 63: 72-74, 1950.
16. Idem. Uncontrollable hives (treated by a synthetic adrenal-cortex compound). *Can. Med. Assoc. J.* 63: 292-293, 1950.
17. Sugarman, H. and Baltzan, D.M. Mucosal respiratory syndrome. *Can. Med. Assoc. J.* 66: 68-69, 1952.
18. Idem. Anginal syndromes. *Can. Med. Assoc. J.* 73: 396-399, 1957.
19. Idem. An Introduction to medicine in Russia (abridged from the annual St. Paul's staff Christmas address). *Can. Med. Assoc. J.* 76: 242-243, 1957.
20. Idem. and Maddin, W. Stuart. Medicine in China. *Can. Med. Assoc. J.* 93: 1118-1122, 1965.
21. Idem. After the six-day war comes an atmosphere of tranquillity. *Saskatoon Star-Phoenix* August 31, 1967.
22. Idem. C.M.A. Forum. An impediment to the evolutionary process. *Can. Med. Assoc. J.* 107: 667-668, 1972.
23. Idem. Telemetric medical services can provide a voice in the wilderness. *Can. Med. Assoc. J.* 112: 1138-1141, 1975.

Notes

Chapter 1

1. Royal Commission on Health Services. Ottawa 1964. Catalogue No. Z1-1961/3-1. Three of the seven commissioners were doctors.
2. The Course of Medicare Programs, a lecture delivered at a seminar for a national group of medical students in hospital administration, University of Saskatchewan, Saskatoon, 3 June 1965. *Diefenbaker Papers,* archives, Diefenbaker Centre, University of Saskatchewan, Saskatoon.
3. Interview with Emmett Hall in Saskatoon, 15 April 1992.
4. Gruending, Dennis *Emmett Hall: Establishment Radical, a biography of Emmett Hall.* Macmillan Canada 1985.
5. Ibid. p. 95.

Chapter 2

1. Memories of a Western Canadian Jewish *Peneep,* by Jacob Baltzan, Lipton, Saskatchewan, 1904-1908. Baltzan family records.
2. Interview with Rose (Collins) Rudd in Saskatoon, August, 1993.
3. Obituary, by Harold Segall, MD, Canadian Medical Association Journal, Aug. 1, 1983, pp. 294-295.
4. Interview with Lorna Whelan in Saskatoon, July, 1993.

5. Interview with Marc Baltzan in Saskatoon, March, 1993.
6. Baltzan story . . . farm boy climbs to fame and fortune, Saskatoon Star-Phoenix, Sept. 28, 1974.
7. Obituary, by Harold Segall, MD, Canadian Medical Association Journal, Aug. 1, 1983, pp. 294-295.

Chapter 3

1. Baltzan story . . . farm boy climbs to fame and fortune, by Pat O'Dwyer, Saskatoon Star-Phoenix, Sept. 28, 1974.
2. Interview with Rose (Collins) Rudd in Saskatoon, August, 1993.
3. Ibid.
4. Ibid.
5. Interview in Saskatoon with John Chrones, March, 1994.
6. Interview with Harold Sugarman, MD in Saskatoon August, 1993.
7. Ibid.
8. Interview with Emmett Hall April 15, 1992 in Saskatoon.
9. Interview with Lorna Whelan in Saskatoon, July, 1993.
10. Ibid.
11. Interview with Marc Baltzan in Saskatoon, March, 1993.

Chapter 4

1. see Appendix 2 no. 1
2. see Appendix 2 no. 2
3. see Appendix 2 no. 3
4. In 1912 Kinnier Wilson (1877-1937) described the condition which bears his name. In 1861 F.T. Frerichs had described a similar condition of simultaneous degeneration of the liver and lenticular nucleus of the brain but neither he nor Wilson recognized it as a disorder of copper metabolism. By the time of Baltzan's report in 1936 the essential characteristic of Wilson's disease was known: Haurowitz (Z. *physiol. Chemie, 1990,* 72, 1930) had demonstrated excessive amounts of copper in the liver and brain. It is not clear from Baltzan's article if he was aware of the connection between abnormal copper storage and hepato-lenticular degeneration (Wilson's disease). Until the report of Uzman and Denny-Brown (Amer. J. med. sci.*215* 599, 1948) in the English language literature reviewed all published cases to date, it is unlikely the implication of copper would have been widely recognized.

5. see Appendix 2 no. 5
6. see Appendix 2 no. 6
7. see Appendix 2 no. 7
8. see Appendix 2 no. 8
9. see Appendix 2 no. 9
10. see Appendix 2 no. 11
11. see Appendix 2 no. 10
12. see Appendix 2 no. 13
13. see Appendix 2 no. 14
14. see Appendix 2 no. 15
15. see Appendix 2 no. 16
16. see Appendix 2 no. 18
17. see Appendix 2 no. 22
18. see Appendix 2 no. 23

Chapter 5

1. Interview with Marc Baltzan in Saskatoon March 1993.
2. Interview with Harold Sugarman in Saskatoon August 1993.
3. Kidney transplant waiting list leaps 40 per cent since 1989. *Saskatoon StarPhoenix,* Jan. 4, 1994.
4. Interview with Marc Baltzan in Saskatoon March 1993.

Chapter 6

1. Spencer, Dick. *Trumpets and Drums: Diefenbaker on the Campaign Trail.* Vancouver: Douglas & McIntyre 1994.

Chapter 7

1. The Saskatoon StarPhoenix of 20 October 1958.
2. see Appendix 2 no. 19
3. Interview with Marc Baltzan in Saskatoon March 1993.
4. see Appendix 2 no. 20

Chapter 8

1. Interview with Dr. Ernie Baergen.
2. Saskatchewan Medical Association files.
3. Letters Patent of Continuance granted by the Minister of Consumer and Corporate Affairs, 1971. In: Shephard, D.A.E., *The Royal College of Physicians and Surgeons of Canada 1960-1980. The pursuit of Unity.*

Ottawa, The Royal College of Physicians and Surgeons of Canada. 1985. p. 439.

Chapter 9

1. Records of Congregation Agudas Israel, Saskatchewan Archives, University of Saskatchewan.
2. Clubb, S.P. *Our Story: 75 Years of Caring: St. Paul's Grey Nun's of Saskatoon*. Modern Press 1981.

Chapter 10

1. Mendel, F.S. *The Book and Life of a Little Man*. Toronto. Macmillan Canada, 1972.
2. Interview with Marc and Richard Baltzan in Saskatoon, May, 1984.
3. Thomas, Dylan. Do Not Go Gentle into That Good Night. In *Collected Poems*. J.M. Dent 1988.

Index